Ethical Principle in Catholic Health Care

Ethical Principle in Catholic Health Care

Edward James Furton, M.A., Ph.D.
Editor

Veronica McLoud Dort, M.T.S.
Assistant Editor

Short Essays in Catholic Medical Ethics
Volume I
The National Catholic Bioethics Center

Nihil Obstat: Rev. Romanus Cessario, O.P., S.T.D.
Imprimatur: Bernard Cardinal Law
Date: October 20, 1999

The Nihil Obstat and Imprimatur are a declaration that a book or pamphlet is considered to be free from doctrinal or moral error.
It is not implied that those who granted the Nihil Obstat and Imprimatur agree with the contents, opinions, or statements expressed therein.

Cover Design:
Thomas Gannoe

Library of Congress Cataloging-in-Publication Data

Ethical principle in Catholic health care / Edward James Furton, editor ; Veronica McLoud Dort, assistant editor.
p. cm. -- (Short essays in Catholic medical ethics ; v. 1)
Includes index.
ISBN 0-935372-42-3
1. Medical ethics. 2. Christian ethics--Catholic authors. 3. Medicine--Religious aspects--Catholic Church. I. Furton, Edward James. II. Dort, Veronica McLoud III. Series.

R725.56 .E84 1999
174'.2--dc21

99-051420

Preface

In the 2000th Year of our Lord, the monthly bulletin of The National Catholic Bioethics Center, *Ethics & Medics*, enters its twenty-fifth continuous year of publication. So it seems an auspicious time to begin a new series of volumes that present to our readers the best and most important articles that have appeared in its pages. This humble two-page publication, with its distinctive blue design and simple lines, has published original articles from authors as diverse as college students and Nobel Prize winners, from nurses, counselors, and physicians, from distinguished clergymen, academics, and scientific researchers. *Ethics & Medics* has found more than its niche in the field of medical-morality and bioethics; it has become a touchstone for the best Catholic thinking in the field.

What would appear to be the most serious disadvantage of writing for *Ethics & Medics* turns out, in fact, to be its most distinctive advantage. Our authors must state in a brief compass of approximately 1,600 words the essence of their views. This forces writers to come directly (and thankfully) to the point. Though we occasionally publish an essay that spans two issues, the need for compression gives *Ethics & Medics* a straightforwardness that corresponds to a world in which time appears to flow at an increasingly rapid pace. Our readers are the busy people who want to stay in touch with present debate among physicians, scientists, church leaders, ethicists, and theologians about pressing moral issues in the health and life sciences.

The brevity and directness of those essays is present here in a volume of best essays that gives the reader an easy entry into the most essential features of the Catholic approach to medical ethics.

The National Catholic Bioethics Center is known for its fidelity to the Magisterium of the Roman Catholic Church and for its unwillingness to publish or promote ideas that are contrary to magisterial teachings. In the areas of medical ethics and bioethics, however, there are many moral issues that remain unresolved. Not all of the articles in these volumes will please all readers. When moral and theological opinion is divided, this series will present both sides of the issue. Supporters of The National Center sometimes express frustration over this lack of resolution, but it does not fall to any institution short of the Holy See itself to make the final determination in these matters. We serve the Church best when we provide a forum in which moral debate can flourish and so help provide the Church with the materials necessary to reflect upon and eventually resolve these issues.

Today The National Center faces an enormous increase in the number of moral challenges that confront us as Americans and as Catholics. In many ways, the Catholic Church is a greater sign of contradiction today than she ever was in the past. Defense of the non-profit and Christ-centered character of health care puts her at odds with a profit-conscious corporate culture. Opposition to abortion, physician-assisted suicide, sterilization, and other intrinsically immoral practices puts her out of step with the supposedly more enlightened and progressive thinkers in America. Equally distinctive, the Catholic Church brings a philosophical tradition with principles as old as Aristotle to contemporary moral analysis of the most advanced medical and scientific technologies. The high regard among Catholics for the "autonomous enterprise" of reason, to use John Paul II's eloquent phrase [*Fides et ratio*, #75], has given the Catholic faith a unique standing among Christians—and indeed, among all religious faiths throughout the world. Our elaborate educational system, our many colleges and universities, our many newspapers, journals, and wire services, and most importantly for the readers of this volume, our extensive system of hospitals and other health care facilities, all display the unique desire among Catholics to work with faith and reason.

This particular volume of essays focuses on the broadest themes. Essays have been chosen with an eye to laying out what it means to offer health care in a Catholic setting, what challenges face Catholic ethicists and health care providers, and what tools and intellectual resources are available to us from our tradition to address these challenges. Future volumes will address more specific and practical issues in the provision of health care and the problems that arise from the dizzying advance of medical science and technology.

The U.S. bishops' *Ethical and Religious Directives for Catholic Health Care Services* [1995] is often cited in this volume. That work is a brief exposition of Catholic principles that govern all Catholic health care providers and Catholic health care institutions in the United States. As such, it is a vital document for anyone who would seek to understand the Catholic outlook on health care. The directives are not yet in their final form—and indeed, they never will be, for they are subject to regular revision at the direction of the U.S. bishops, as the need arises. With the increasing pace of change in the field of health care, we can expect constant revisions in the future. Copies of the current edition of the *Directives* are available from the United States Conference of Catholic Bishops in Washington, D.C., or from The National Center.

Edward J. Furton, M.A., Ph.D.
Editor, *Ethics & Medics*

Moral Theory in the Catholic Tradition

Catholic Care

Human Dignity and Health Care 5
John M. Haas, S.T.L., Ph.D.

Catholic Identity in Health Care 9
Daniel P. Maher, Ph.D.

The Moral Status of Compassion 13
Edmund D. Pellegrino, M.D.

Moral Doctrine

Role of the Magisterium in Christian Life 19
William E. May, Ph.D.

What Is Conscience Anyway? 23
Rev. David N. Beauregard, O.M.V., Ph.D.

On Imposing Our Morality on Others 27
Joseph Boyle, Ph.D.

Law and Virtue

Natural Law and Human Virtue 33
Russell Hittinger, Ph.D.

Virtue or Obligation in Catholic Ethics? 37
Rev. David N. Beauregard, O.M.V., Ph.D.

Human Freedom and Natural Law 41
Rev. Servais Théodore Pinckaers, O.P.

Principles of Catholic Bioethics

Christ-Centered

Christian Anthropology and Happiness 49
Ralph McInerny, Ph.D.

Christ as Moral Example and Teacher 53
Peter Kreeft, Ph.D.

The Mystery of Suffering 57
Rev. David N. Beauregard, O.M.V., Ph.D.

Reflective Action

Stewardship, Dominion, and Autonomy 63
Rev. Germain Kopaczynski, OFM Conv., Ph.D., S.T.D.

The Error of Proportionalism 67
Janet E. Smith, Ph.D.

Intention and the Object of Choice 73
David M. Gallagher, Ph.D.

The Principled Decision

The Principle of Double Effect 81
Peter J. Cataldo, Ph.D.

The Totality and Integrity of the Body 85
John M. Haas, S.T.L., Ph.D.

Ordinary versus Extraordinary Means 89
Rev. Russell E. Smith, S.T.D.

The Catholic Health Care Institution

Service to the Community

Not-for-Profit Catholic Health Care 97
Rev. Michael D. Place, S.T.D.

Technological Achievement or Patient Health? 101
Charles E. Cavagnaro III, M.D.

Establishing a Hospital Ethics Committee 105
Daniel O'Brien, Ph.D.

Respect for the Patient

Confidentiality and Truth-Telling 111
Charles E. Cavagnaro III, M.D.

Justice as a Social Virtue 115
Theodore P. Rebard, Ph.D.

Human Experimentation and Research 119
Rev. Albert S. Moraczewski, O.P., Ph.D., S.T.M.

Engaging the Public

Is the Written Law Ethical? 125
Stephen M. Krason, J.D., Ph.D.

Catholic Hospitals and Abortion Physicians 129
Sr. Jean DeBlois, C.S.J., Ph.D.

Individual and Corporate Cooperation 133
Rev. Russell E. Smith, S.T.D.

Growth in the Market

Avoiding Formal Cooperation in Health Care Alliances 139
The National Catholic Bioethics Center

Models of Collaborative Arrangements 147
Peter J. Cataldo, Ph.D.

The Philadelphia Protocol for Collaborative Relationships . . 151
The Archdiocese of Philadelphia

Five Principles for Collaborative Arrangements 155
The National Catholic Bioethics Center

Index 159

Moral Theory in the Catholic Tradition

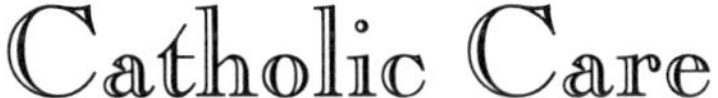

Catholic Care

Human Dignity and Health Care

At the heart of the *Ethical and Religious Directives for Catholic Health Care Services* (National Conference of Catholic Bishops [1995]), the governing document for Catholic health care in the United States, is the recognition of the inviolable dignity of each and every human being. It is love for the suffering individual that has drawn Catholics into health care and restrains them from ever doing anything that would harm or violate that individual in any way. At the very beginning of the document, the *Directives* state: "First, Catholic health care ministry is rooted in a commitment to promote and defend human dignity; this is the foundation of its concern to respect the sacredness of every human life from the moment of conception until death" (Introduction to Part One).

The Meaning of Dignity

There is surely no lack of assertions of the dignity of the human person in our day. In fact, those who would advocate euthanasia and physician-assisted suicide do so with the claim that it is precisely such actions that would be in harmony with the dignity of the suffering person. The advocates of euthanasia call for "death with dignity." Problems arise, however, when one attempts to understand what is meant by the human dignity lauded by so many today. By their own stated positions and advocacy of certain social policies, "human dignity" would seem to refer, in large part, to the ability of an individual to do whatever he may feel inclined to do. Those who have such an understanding of human dignity would naturally become quite dismayed, in fact, perhaps "dismayed unto death," if they would find themselves seriously disabled as the result of an accident or illness and incapable of doing what they might feel inclined to do. Indeed, such a life might well be "not worth living" in their estimation. But is the ability to do whatever one feels inclined to do actually the criterion by which human dignity is judged?

Within the Catholic tradition, dignity refers to the excellence or nobility of the person. Even in our day, no one is judged excellent or noble simply for doing whatever he may feel inclined to do—such as drinking to the point of intoxication or lying to another so as to gain an unjust advantage. Dignity is still associated with some understanding of goodness or excellence. But how can a newborn or a patient in a coma be considered good if they are unable to engage in good and noble actions? So the dignity inherent in every human being must have a source other than the noble deeds performed by the individual: there is also a dignity that is given or bestowed, not gained.

It must be stated most emphatically that every human person enjoys an inherent dignity that must be respected and in no way violated, even when such an individual may not be fully competent or may have even acted in evil ways. Indeed, the inviolability of the human person has led to the Church's insistence on moral absolutes. There are some actions that may never be done under any circumstances. Performing these actions would constitute a violation of the person's dignity: the dignity of the one against whom the action is directed *as well as the one performing the action.*

The Source of Dignity

The question may be asked, from where does the dignity of the individual human person derive? A person's dignity is inherent, a permanent and inseparable quality, yet this quality is not any more necessary than is the existence of the person and does not explain itself. No one necessarily exists. Furthermore, no one enjoys such self-evident excellence or nobility that he would naturally elicit awe and reverence in the other to such a degree that the other would not even contemplate violating such goodness. The excellence of each individual human being is then to be understood as fundamentally participatory, i.e., it shares in that alone which is of its nature excellent and noble and true and beautiful: God Himself. The *Directives* make this clear: "The dignity of human life flows from creation in the image of God (Gen. 1:26), from redemption by Jesus Christ (Eph.1:10; 1 Tim. 2:4–6), and from our common destiny to share a life with God beyond all corruption (1 Cor.15:42–57)" (Introduction to Part Two).

The reality of human dignity is also seen in the first quotation above from the *Directives*,which speaks of "the sacredness of every human life." In the last analysis, the sacred is properly an attribute of God alone. "I the Lord your God am holy" (Lev. 19:2). Persons, places, things, and times become holy when they have been touched by God. The "sacredness of every human life" is a participatory sacredness. "To me, therefore, you shall be sacred; for I the Lord am sacred" (Lev. 20:26).

Morality vs. Legalism

The Catholic moral tradition has always taught that there are some actions that must never be done because they are intrinsically disordered, i.e., they do fundamental violence to the sacredness of human life. People usually lose sight of the relationship that exists between that which is judged to be morally illicit and the violence committed against some good of the human person. It appears to many people that the Church's judgment that certain actions are immoral is little more than an arbitrary expression of distaste, or of a decision to apply some willful strictures against the pursuit of human happiness in order to maintain control over Church members.

Tubal ligations and vasectomies, which have been and will be consistently forbidden in Catholic health facilities, strike some as having no more relevance to human goodness and human happiness than eating meat on Fridays, which was once forbidden by the Church. However, the difference is that the one prohibition (against eating meat on Friday) was merely a disciplinary one, whereas the other prohibition (against direct sterilizations) cautions against actions which would directly violate individuals in the very core of their being. In the minds of Catholics, actions such as, for example, *in vitro* fertilization or artificial insemination are not wrong because they have been forbidden by Church authorities. Rather, they have been forbidden in Catholic health facilities because they are wrong and do violence to the dignity of the persons involved.

In the *Summa contra Gentiles* St. Thomas Aquinas says that God is offended by us—not when we violate His commandments—but when we act against our own good. The Ten Commandments were given to us to keep us from acting against our own good! This is precisely why the *Directives* were given to us. They were drawn up for no other reason than to express the Church's solicitude for our vulnerability to being used by others.

A legalistic attitude is surely the principal reason that Catholic moral teachings, and consequently the *Directives*, are misunderstood. It would come as a surprise to many, Catholics as well as non-Catholics, that sin is defined in the *Catechism of the Catholic Church* (see n. 1849) not principally as a violation of God's commandments, but rather as an offense against reason and truth! In other words, sin is an offense against that unique capacity of human beings, their reason, which is the highest mark of their dignity and the very image of God within them.

It must be said that the only thing that will truly violate the dignity of an individual is sin. This is one reason why the *Directives* prohibit certain procedures in Catholic health facilities; they have the defect of sinfulness and therefore are simply beneath the dignity of human beings who are created in the image and likeness of God.

As stated repeatedly in the *Directives*, Catholic health care facilities are concerned with the good of the whole person, physical, emotional, and spiritual. But one of these goods cannot be arbitrarily chosen to the detriment of the other. Indeed there is a hierarchy of goods, so that one ought to be ready to sacrifice a physical good if pursuing it would mean violating a spiritual good. Nothing can come before our relationship with God, and the only thing that can impede that relationship is sin. To paraphrase Our Lord: *What would it profit a man to gain the best physical health in the world but to lose his soul?*

Dignity and Moral Principles

It is because of the Catholic Church's commitment to the inviolable dignity of each human being that she insists upon such patient rights as informed consent and autonomy, the right of all not to be arbitrarily denied access to health care, especially those who are weak and vulnerable. It is because of the Church's desire to avoid violating human dignity that her moral tradition has developed such refined tools of philosophical and moral reflection as the principle of double effect and principles governing material cooperation in evil, or distinctions between the directly and indirectly voluntary, or between ordinary and extraordinary means of preserving life. Part Three of the *Directives* spells out in considerable detail some of the implications of respecting the dignity of the individual person. Directive 23 states: "The inherent dignity of the human person must be respected and protected regardless of the nature of the person's health problem or social status. The respect for human dignity extends to all persons who are served by Catholic health care."

Health Subordinated to Human Dignity

The dignity of the human person rests in his being created in the image and likeness of God. A direct, willful violation of any person is in some sense an act of sacrilege, doing violence to the image of God and to that degree it expresses contempt for the person's Creator. This realization should help health care professionals, and even clergy, keep health care in perspective; the victory over death has already been won by Christ and will never be won by medical researchers. But all must still undergo death as punishment for sin before entering into life everlasting. A "life with God beyond all corruption" (Introduction to Part Two) must be the goal and aspiration of all. The only thing that would prevent us from enjoying such a life is sin, not blocked arteries. Consequently anything done to preserve or restore our health must not do violence to our inherent dignity. A faithful interpretation and application of the *Directives* will at least help us maintain the disposition and attitude toward the recipients of health care that are truly in harmony with their dignity—and will help health care workers maintain their own dignity.

John M. Haas, S.T.L., Ph.D.
President
The National Catholic Bioethics Center
Boston, Massachusetts

Catholic Identity in Health Care

Is there a place for Catholicism in the health care field? In a word, No. There are, rather, *places*, a number of different ways to exercise Catholic belief within health care. Sitting at the bedside of a dying man because in him you see Christ is not the same thing as reading an MRI or taking part in a hospital's strategic planning meeting. Yet all can be manifestations of the Church's healing ministry. If we fail to attend to the differences among these activities, we might come to believe that Catholic health care is simpler than it is. We might try to assimilate all its forms to the image of the Good Samaritan, for example. This happens in some simplistic characterizations, such as, "Catholic institutions offer health care for the love of God, without any question of return." Such pious but naive claims are likely to insult someone who has just received a bill for a stay in a Catholic hospital. Trying to make all of Catholic health care sound as charitable as only some of it is opens the door to charges of hypocrisy.

Catholic Health Care Is Not Free Care

Catholic health care is charitable indeed, but not all of it is charitable in the same way. "Charity" has more than one meaning, and the most important meaning is not financial. For this reason, the identifying mark of Catholic health care is not that it is provided without regard for the patient's ability to pay. The matter is more complicated, and it would be wrong to believe that health care is Catholic because it is free. This confusion would suggest that only *unreimbursed* care counts as *Catholic* health care. The Catholicity of health care is not reducible to how money is managed.

The delivery of health care in any form requires money, and religious sponsors of health care need a source of money for the good they do. Even when a health care apostolate takes a form that is not expensive, those who provide their time and attention can do so only because they are free from the need to provide for themselves. Tending to someone else presupposes that one's own needs are already met. The financial requirements for providing state-of-the-art health care are monumentally high. In order to secure adequate resources, sponsors must serve not only the poor, but also those who can pay. Payers are not only individuals, but also government agencies and corporations such as HMOs. Because they pay the bills, governmental and corporate payers—whose own concerns may be hostile to, or perhaps sympathetic to, but more likely indifferent to Catholicism—have power to shape how providers deliver health care. Catholic sponsors are unable to operate entirely on their own terms because they must face fiscal necessities.

The Survival of Catholic Identity

Catholic health care providers, like all providers, are adapting to social, legal, and economic pressures. They are transforming themselves to such a degree that some question whether their Catholicity can survive the metamorphosis. Behind this question there lies another question, which asks whether Catholic health care can survive at all.

When people discuss Catholic identity in health care, they concentrate on the minimum or *sine qua non* that health care must be in order to call itself Catholic. Catholic health care typically means, minimally, nontransgression of the prohibitions in the *Ethical and Religious Directives for Catholic Health Care Services* (National Conference of Catholic Bishops [1995]). The question of Catholic identity then becomes a question of whether innovations in medicine and in health care delivery systems are permissible under the current *Directives*.

It is, of course, important not to violate the *Ethical and Religious Directives*, but this merely negative criterion does not display what being Catholic contributes nor why there should be any Catholic presence in health care. Without clearly understanding the contribution of Catholicism to health care, whether a given procedure or arrangement is consistent with Catholic teaching loses its proper context. Lack of self-understanding could reduce the Catholicity of the provider to a limiting factor, boundary lines outside which one must not stray.

Catholic belief and teaching can contribute far more than this to health care. Specifically, the Church claims to have a true and comprehensive account of the meaning and goal of human life. Because of what the Church teaches about the origin and destiny of human life, many people have been inspired to bear witness to this teaching through health care as an apostolate. The Church can show the place of bodily health within the horizon provided by a revealed teaching about the meaning of life. This teaching is needed because our world is fundamentally uncertain about the purpose or meaning of life—an uncertainty that arises in part because the science we accept as the most authoritative form of knowledge tells us nothing about what is good. We recognize experts in physics, astronomy, medicine, etc., but there are no commonly recognized experts in the knowledge of what is good. In particular, the science of medicine, which might be considered the science of human life, despite continual progress, is and will always be unable to answer two fundamental questions: What is a human being? What is a good human being? These are not medical or scientific questions in the sense in which medicine is a science. Consequently, medicine is helpless to answer them.

Guiding the Hand of Medicine

Medicine is knowledge of *how* to maintain health, not knowledge of what is the good. Medicine tells us how to relieve this symptom or how to cure that disease. It shows us how to conceive a child and how not to. Medicine is, however, incapable of telling us which of these alternatives is good. Health is good, but not the only good, and medical science does not tell us how to rank health relative to other goods. Most of us recognize that there are other things more important than health and even life, things for which we would risk our health or sacrifice our lives, such as family, justice, or freedom. We would condemn someone who would stop at nothing in order to preserve his own life.

Medicine is expertise in how to produce health, but the knowledge for producing health is also the knowledge for producing disease and death. Medicine tells us what dosage of a drug will preserve life and *simultaneously* it tells us what dosage will end life. Every art has this dual capacity: If it is necessary to demolish an old building, architects know where to place the charges to cause it to collapse into itself. Auto mechanics best know how to disable a car.

Medical science, then, confers tremendous power to heal or to harm, but it does not confer wisdom in the use of that power. The practice of medicine requires guidance concerning how and to what purposes its knowledge should be used. Historically, the Hippocratic Oath and other professional codes helped to ensure that medical knowledge be used in acceptable ways. These codes stating the ends of medicine are not themselves established by medical experiments, but by moral or political views of one sort or another. Medicine is never morally neutral, whether it is aware of its moral presuppositions or not. This country is now debating which ends medicine should serve. Previously, we thought it should serve life and health above all, but the argument that medicine might take life in order to limit suffering is now gaining popular acceptance.

Even if it is agreed that life and health are the goods to be preserved, it must still be decided which means to these ends are good or bad. A couple wants a child, but is having difficulty conceiving. Some techniques produce multiple pregnancies and call for "selective reduction," some produce a child in a laboratory, and some call for the use of surrogates. Medicine can judge which are technically effective and what the attendant risks are, but it cannot say whether and at what price it is good to attain a child. Adoption and kidnapping are also ways of securing a child, but medical knowledge, as such, does not judge the moral goodness or badness of any of these methods. Medical knowledge judges only the effectiveness of the medical means for achieving the desired goal.

To be sure, a physician is also a moral agent who judges his or her own actions as good or bad. Physicians are morally responsible for their practice of medicine and often turn to their own moral principles in their medical decisions. Nevertheless, these are moral judgments made on moral, not medical grounds.

The point is not that physicians are amoral or evil unless the Church controls health care, but that it is easy to overlook that the *goodness* of the ends or goals of medicine is not determined by medical science. We often take for granted that physicians are decent human beings promoting life and health, until someone out of the ordinary appears (e.g., Jack Kevorkian). The vast majority of physicians may be morally exemplary human beings, but medical science itself offers no wisdom about the meaning of life and death nor about the place of health in the good life. Catholic teaching about human life shows the place that medicine should occupy in a good life.

The Catholic Aim for Health Care

Catholic health care takes many forms, and misunderstanding some of its forms may give people working in Catholic facilities a bad conscience. Some who are pressured to meet financial demands as part of their job spend so much time and energy trying to make or save money that they suspect their institution does not really serve the poor, but only its financial welfare. Others may believe that following the *Ethical and Religious Directives* constitutes bad medicine or at least a failure to meet urgent health needs, perhaps because they consider the *Directives* distorted by "archaic" sexual teachings. Both these attitudes display a lack of understanding of Catholic health care. First, Catholic health care is not only for the poor, because the teaching about life is true also of the paying sick, the employees, and even of competitors. Second, the ethical prohibitions in Catholic teaching do not conflict with the good of the patient, but promote the use of medicine in the best interests of human life.

Catholicism provides an answer to how medicine should use its power. Because many people believe what the Church teaches—that each human life is created in the image of God—they have been inspired to provide the healing benefits of the highest quality of medical care to those who suffer from all manner of illnesses. Some people actually believe that this teaching is Good News and that medicine practiced in the light of this teaching is the very best health care available. They are not ashamed that they cannot provide an abortion to a woman who has been raped; they do not find it absurd to teach teenagers about abstinence rather than distribute condoms; and they do not harbor desires to perform tubal ligations. For these faithful believers, the Church's teaching does not function as a leash, but as a light guiding the way to the proper and legitimate uses of medicine in the best interests of human life. Rather than leaving medicine to be driven by contemporary social currents, the Church, through her moral teaching, illluminates the course medicine should follow; it falls to believers and others of good will to take up the oars.

Daniel P. Maher, Ph.D.
Assistant Professor of Philosophy
The Catholic University of America
Washington, D.C.

The Moral Status of Compassion

Compassion is a word used frequently in the moral lexicons of Catholic Christians and secular humanists. Both invoke it to support the actions they deem morally valid in response to human suffering, especially when it involves the origins, sustenance, and ending of human life. But there is a significant difference in the moral weight each gives to compassion and the way each responds to its urgings.

On the one hand, we have the inspiring meditation on human life in Pope John Paul II's encyclical *Evangelium vitae*. The Pope's words are filled with Christ's compassion for the sick, the dying, the unborn, and the aged. He calls us to be compassionate as Christ was compassionate: to relieve suffering, but always with respect for the inviolable sanctity and dignity of all human life, however fragile, young or old, sick or well. On the other hand, there is the claim of secular humanists that they are the possessors of true compassion for the suffering. For them, suffering is the greatest evil, and the relief of suffering, the greatest good. Compassion justifies taking the life of the sufferer, helping him to take his own life, or taking the lives of others to relieve suffering, for example, by aborting the unwanted or genetically imperfect fetus, creating embryos for research purposes, and using aborted embryos for tissue transplantation.

Between the Christian and secular interpretations of compassion, there is a grave moral and conceptual dissonance. For the secularist, the sentiment of compassion has moral weight of its own. It is, itself, a virtue which entails relief of pain and suffering as the major end of moral life. For the Christian, sentiment cannot function as a reason for moral choice. Sentiment is not a virtue unless ordered by reason, and suffering has a definite meaning in human lives. As *Evangelium vitae* so richly attests, the resulting dichotomy leads in opposite directions—to a "new culture of life" on the one hand, or to the culture of death on the other.

Compassion—The Sentiment and the Virtue

Christians and secular humanists both begin at the same place. Each recognizes the ubiquity of the *feeling* of compassion, which is an emotion experienced by all but the most depraved humans in the presence of another person's suffering. Thus, compassion is an affective state: feeling something of another's suffering, suffering along with another, and making another's suffering at least partially our own. Compassion differs from mercy, which inclines to kindness where severity might be deserved, and from pity, which means feeling sorry for another. Neither mercy nor pity entails the intimate sharing of pain and suffering encompassed by compassion.

Although both *feel* compassion, Christians and secular humanists part company when it comes to assessing its moral status, the weight it should carry in justification, and whether it is a virtue in itself. For the Christian, the sentiment of compassion may be laudable, but it is not self-justifying. It needs to be under the control of reason if it is to be a virtue and not degenerate into vice. For the secularist, the sentiment itself is a warrant for action, and in itself is a virtue to which reason can add little.

The Secular Religion of Compassion

The modern secular meaning of compassion arose with the sentimentalist philosophers of the eighteenth century who assumed a moral sense that made humans compassionate. Rousseau (1712–1778), for example, thought this natural sentiment was a better guide to virtue than Christian teaching. David Hume (1711–1776) held that reason should be a slave to the passions and is, of itself, incapable of motivating moral acts. They, and others, offer in place of Christianity a substitute natural religion in which original sin is abolished, agreeable and useful sentiments become virtues, and the source of all meaning for suffering is demolished.

In this natural religion, the feeling of compassion is, itself, a virtue without the need for guidance by reason. In that religion, suffering becomes the greatest of evils and its alleviation the greatest human good. This natural religion is the religion of today's conscientious secular humanist. It exalts the sentiment of compassion to a self-justifying principle. As long as a thing is done out of genuine compassion, as long as it "feels good," it is morally good and, even if taken to an extreme, morally requisite. On this view, much of contemporary moral life consists in the relief of suffering— suffering which is meaningless according to the canons of natural religion.

Compassion is torn, therefore, from its roots in the Christian tradition with two results: 1) outside the Christian ethic, the only life worth living is a life without undue suffering; and 2) suffering expands to include every troubling event in life, since someone "suffers" from every perceived deprivation in the quality of the life he or she lives.

In terms of natural religion, to be compassionate is to eliminate suffering by whatever means are available and in whatever sense suffering is interpreted. This has come to entail killing or assisting in the suicide of the chronically ill or comatose adult who does not die easily enough, killing or failing to provide sustenance to the badly handicapped infant whose prospects for a "quality" life are dim, aborting the inconvenient pregnancy, artificially inseminating the infertile woman, "assisting" the death of severely depressed persons whose life has lost its satisfactions, or hastening death for those "suffering" patients too dulled mentally to be able to consent to their own demise.

It is undeniable that all of these persons suffer in one way or another. They elicit our compassion. But compassion torn from its roots in the Christian tradition leads to the Culture of Death. The Catholic novelist Flannery O'Connor said that the logical outcome of tenderness separated from its source in Christ is terror. Compassion is an emotion that itself demands to be served, to have its source removed—the suffering of the observer—as much as the suffering of the patient.

Compassion as a Christian Virtue

When compassion becomes a habitual disposition, a consistent willingness to share in, and to relieve, another's suffering, it becomes a character trait. This character trait becomes a virtue when it inclines a person to make good moral choices among the means used to relieve suffering. To make choices, the sentiment of compassion must be ordered by reason to the good for humans. When it is ordered to the natural good of human life, for example, human fulfillment, it is a natural virtue. When it is ordered to the supernatural ends of human life, then it is infused by charity and becomes a Christian virtue.

For the Christian, compassion in itself, simply as an emotion, is neither a virtue nor a vice. It is not a self-justifying principle. It is the way we choose to act with reference to the emotion that makes it a virtue or a vice (cf. Aristotle, *Nicomachean Ethics,* 1105b 25). Christian compassion reunites the human sentiment of compassion with its source in Christ in his Incarnation. As a virtue, Christian compassion disposes us to do all we can to relieve the natural course of suffering, but only in a way that also helps the sufferer to attain the ultimate good for which humans were created—union with God. To be sure, Christian compassion calls upon us to relieve pain, but also to recognize that suffering comprises more than pain. It calls upon us to discern the many spiritual causes of human suffering—alienation from healthy people, anger with God, feelings of guilt for being a burden to others, shame at one's physical appearance, weakness, and the anguish resulting from avoidance and rejection by the world of the healthy.

Christian compassion recognizes the spiritual crisis at the source of the ethical issues surrounding human life. It cannot respond by elimination of the sufferer. To do so would violate the sanctity of life and the sovereignty of God. Rather, Christian compassion relieves suffering as zealously as does the secular humanist but more effectively within the ethical constraints of natural and divine law. As the *Catechism of the Catholic Church* states, "[C]harity demands beneficence" (n. 1829)—a healing, not a person-eradicating, beneficence.

Christian compassion recognizes charity as the wellspring without which the emotion of compassion can so easily justify the remedy of death and oblivion for any indisposition we take to be suffering. Charitable compassion gives us insight; it enables us to see Christ in our suffering neighbor. Without this insight, we experience the emotion but may not be able to direct it to healing rather than extinguishing the sufferer along with the suffering. Without charity, compassion ceases to be a virtue and becomes a vice that blinds us to the true needs of the suffering person.

The fact that a neighbor suffers is his claim to our compassion—not just the feeling, but the virtue. This insight helps us to avoid the exaggerated pride that can be associated with compassion, making it a self-aggrandizing experience, a way to assuage guilt or to relieve ourselves of the presence of a suffering person whose proximity causes us anguish. To kill the sufferer is to interrupt his or her way of the cross, his or her journey to salvation. It is to frustrate that final abandonment of body and spirit into the will of the Creator.

Christian compassion helps us to see that humans do not lose their dignity because of pain, physical incapacity, helplessness, or disfigurement. When people speak of the loss of dignity of the dying person, they are really talking about their own reaction to the appearance of the sick person. A human being possesses dignity always as a son or daughter of God—that dignity can never be lost. A human death is always the death of a person with dignity.

Compassion for suffering is an emotion felt by all decent human beings. In all conscientious persons, it motivates the desire to alleviate suffering. In this desire, Catholic Christians and secular humanists can agree. But moral choice determines the way this desire is expressed in beneficent action. In each choice, the feeling of compassion becomes subject to reason and revelation. Without these, compassion can become an instrument of death. The only answer to suffering lies in the Gospel of Life. As Pope John Paul II tells us, this is the only antidote to the nihilism, self-delusion, and despair of a society in which oblivion and death are the panaceas for human ills.

Edmund D. Pellegrino, M.D.
John Carroll Professor of Medicine and Medical Ethics
Georgetown University Medical Center
Washington, D.C.

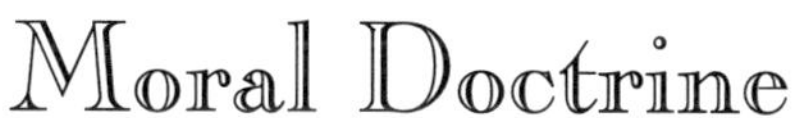

Role of the Magisterium in Christian Life

In his encyclical *Veritatis splendor* (*VS*) Pope John Paul II has well summarized the Church's own self-understanding—as expressed at Vatican II—of the role of the Magisterium in Christian moral life. Therefore, here I will first set forth John Paul II's presentation of this matter (also clearly explained in the *Catechism of the Catholic Church*, nn. 2030–2051). I will then briefly discuss the relationship between the moral teaching proposed by the Magisterium and the conscience of the Catholic. In conclusion, I will discuss the assent due to magisterial moral teachings and the question of their infallibility.

The Moral Authority of the Magisterium

John Paul II reminds us of this more-than-human authority in *Veritatis splendor*. That authority of this kind has been entrusted by Christ to the Apostles and their successors is, the Pope says, "evident from the *living Tradition,* whereby—as the Second Vatican Council teaches—'the Church, in her teaching, life and worship, perpetuates and hands on to every generation all that she is and all that she believes. This Tradition, which comes from the Apostles, progresses within the Church under the assistance of the Holy Spirit' (Vatican II, *Dei Verbum* [*DV*], n. 89)" (*VS*, n. 27).

Continuing, John Paul II goes on to say, "in particular, as the Council affirms, '*the task of authentically interpreting the word of God, whether in its written form or in that of Tradition, has been entrusted only to those charged with the Church's living Magisterium, whose authority is exercised in the name of Jesus Christ*' (*DV*, n.10; emphasis in John Paul II). The Church, in her life and teaching, is thus revealed as 'the pillar and foundation of truth' (1 Tim 3:15), including the truth regarding moral action" (*VS*, n. 27). Moreover, he insists, there is an intimate and inseparable unity between faith and morality inasmuch as the Christian faith "possesses a moral content," giving rise to a "consistent life commitment," requiring those who bear the name Christian to bear "*witness*" before God and man by a living faith that bears fruit in works, "above all those of charity ... manifested and lived in the gift of self, *even to the total gift of self*, like that of Jesus" (nn. 88, 89). Therefore, "no damage must be done to the *harmony between faith and life:* the unity of the Church is damaged not only by Christians who reject or distort the truths of faith but also by those who disregard the moral obligations to which they are called by the Gospel (cf. 1 Cor 5:9–13)" (n. 26).

Moral Teaching and the Conscience of a Catholic

Conscience, in its most precise sense, is a practical judgment that a person makes about what he must do or not do, or one which assesses something he has already done. Indeed, the Catholic tradition has always recognized in the personal judgment of conscience the "*proximate norm of personal morality*," a truth that John Paul II highlights in *VS* (n. 60). Its dignity consists in its capacity to disclose the truth about moral good or evil in the light of God's eternal law, the universal and objective norm of morality (*VS*, nn. 60, 63; Vatican II, *Dignitatis humanae* (*DH*), n. 3; *Gaudium et spes* (*GS*), nn. 16–17). Persons eager to make true moral judgments will, of course, in forming their consciences make every effort to do so well. They will search for the truth and seek to find it from sources where it is most likely to be found.

Thus a Catholic, aware that the Church, speaking through the more-than-human authority vested in the Magisterium, is the "pillar and foundation of truth" (1 Tim 3:15), will be ready to accept the moral teachings of the Magisterium. "In forming their consciences," Vatican II says, "the faithful must pay careful attention to the sacred and certain teaching of the Church. For the Catholic Church is by the will of Christ the teacher of truth. It is her duty to proclaim and teach with authority the truth which is Christ and, at the same time, *to declare and confirm by her authority the principles of the moral order which spring from human nature itself*" (*DH*, n.14, emphasis added).

John Paul II, after citing this passage from Vatican II, goes on to make the following very significant point: "It follows that the authority of the Church, when she pronounces on moral questions, in no way undermines the freedom of conscience of Christians. This is so not only because freedom of conscience is never freedom 'from' the truth but always and only freedom 'in' the truth, but also because *the Magisterium does not bring to the Christian conscience truths which are extraneous to it; rather it brings to light the truths which it ought already to possess, developing them from the starting point of the primordial act of faith*" (*VS*, n. 64, emphasis added). In short, for Catholics the moral teaching of the Church is not an imposition from the outside, but a help for them to make true moral judgments and good moral choices that will enable them to become more fully who they really are: children of God, called to cooperate with Jesus in his redemptive work.

The Assent Due Magisterial Moral Teachings

The Magisterium can propose truths of faith *and* of morals in two ways: infallibly and irreformably, or authoritatively but not irreformably. Truths infallibly proposed by the Magisterium require the assent of faith, whereas truths authoritatively but not irreformably proposed require a "ready and respectful allegiance of mind" and the "loyal submission of the will and intellect" (cf. Vatican II, *Lumen Gentium (LG)*, n. 25).

The Magisterium can propose teachings *infallibly* in two distinct ways. The first is by an extraordinary exercise of its authority through the solemn definitions of ecumenical councils and *ex cathedra* pronouncements of the Roman Pontiff. The second is through the ordinary, day-to-day exercise of the Magisterium when certain conditions are verified. Vatican II clearly articulated these conditions when it affirmed the following: "Although the bishops, taken individually, do not enjoy the privilege of infallibility, they do, however, proclaim *the doctrine of Christ infallibly* on the following conditions: namely, when, even though dispersed throughout the entire world but preserving for all that among themselves and with Peter's successor the bond of communion, in their authoritative teaching concerning matters of faith *or morals*, they are in agreement that a particular teaching is to be held definitively and absolutely. This is still more clearly the case when, assembled in ecumenical council, they are, for the universal Church, teachers of and judges in matters of faith *and morals*, whose judgment must be adhered to with the loyal and obedient assent *of faith*" (*LG*, n. 25, emphasis added; cf. Vatican I, *Dei Filius,* DS 3011).

Although some theologians today claim that the Magisterium *cannot infallibly* propose specific moral norms (e.g., one ought never intentionally to kill innocent human beings; one ought never to have sex outside of marriage), this claim is repudiated by the Magisterium itself (Congregation for the Doctrine of the Faith, *Instruction on the Ecclesial Vocation of the Theologian*, n. 16; Vatican I, *Dei Filius*, DS 3005), and the reasons alleged to support this claim have been shown by competent theologians to be utterly specious (see, e.g., Germain Grisez, *The Way of the Lord Jesus*: *Christian Moral Principles* [Chicago: Franciscan Herald Press, 1983], ch. 36).

Moreover, it was the common understanding of all Catholic theologians prior to Vatican II that the core of Catholic moral teaching, as set forth in its understanding of the precepts of the Decalogue, had been infallibly taught by the Magisterium in its ordinary, day-to-day teaching and therefore required from the faithful the assent of faith (see, e.g., Karl Rahner, *Nature and Grace: Dilemmas in the Modern Church* (London: Sheed & Ward, 1963), 51–52). Nothing taught by Vatican II provides any ground for repudiating this common understanding. Rather, as the citation already given about the infallibility of the bishops united with the pope in their everyday teaching under certain conditions testifies, the teaching of Vatican II confirms it.

Although John Paul II does not explicitly claim, in *Veritatis splendor*, that he is infallibly proposing the truth that there are intrinsically evil acts and, corresponding to them, moral absolutes, he nonetheless explicitly affirms that his teaching on this matter—which simply reaffirms the constant Tradition of the Church—is the teaching of the Scriptures (nn. 78–83) and part of divine revelation. It follows that his teaching in this encyclical on intrinsically evil acts and moral absolutes is a truth demanding from every Catholic the assent of faith. What well-instructed Catholic can ever think that intentionally killing the innocent, having sex outside of marriage, or perjuring oneself on the witness stand could possibly be compatible with life in Christ and with a commitment to participate in his redemptive work?

Moral teaching proposed authoritatively but not irreformably by the Magisterium requires from all Catholics, including popes, bishops, theologians, and the ordinary man and woman, a loyal submission of will and intellect. While it may be permissible, under specific conditions, to raise questions about these teachings and to *suspend* intellectual assent from them—and the Magisterium itself explicitly acknowledges that this can be legitimate (see *Instruction on the Ecclesial Vocation of the Theologian*, nn. 24–31)—it is never right for a Catholic to *dissent from* these teachings, to declare that they are erroneous and that a Catholic is at liberty to set them aside and act contrary to them. This is to damage the unity of the Church and arrogantly to usurp the authority given by Christ to the Magisterium.

William E. May, Ph.D.
Michael J. McGivney Professor of Moral Theology
John Paul II Institute for Studies on Marriage and Family
Washington, D.C.

What Is Conscience Anyway?

Perhaps the most important term in modern moral discourse is conscience. "What my conscience tells me" is considered something absolutely personal, definitive, and beyond criticism. It is conceived of largely as a righteous, often self-righteous, opposition to authority. As Cardinal Ratzinger has observed, in reaction to a pre-Vatican II morality of authority, conscience has become "the bulwark of freedom" opposing "the encroachments of authority" (*Conscience and Truth* [Braintree, MA: Pope John Center, 1991], 1). It is the perfect moral instrument for liberal democracies, in which the autonomous individual, in being true to himself, makes moral decisions in isolation from society, from authority—and from truth. The somewhat arresting irony is that in such a context, conscience becomes the absolute expression of a relativistic subjectivity.

Conscience and Truth

From this rootedness in subjectivity arises what *Veritatis splendor* (*VS*) has indicated is the crucial problem: the relation of conscience to truth (nn. 54–64). Even if I believe I am doing the right thing in all good conscience, if my conscience is in fact erroneous, if it is not rooted in the truth, then I myself am at risk (see *VS* 63). I must use my intelligence to perceive what is truly good, not what is expedient or apparently good because of the pressure of my personal circumstances or personal bias. For example, I may believe that homosexuality or contraception or abortion are good forms of behavior. But that is a misperception that will not change reality, or absolve me of the real effects of my actions, which in the case of these three forms of behavior may result in AIDS or a coronary embolism or post-abortion depression. Thus, in the interests of human flourishing and my own good, it is essential that conscience be founded on intelligent perception, indeed that it be rooted in reality and truth. To found it on mere will, on blind choice, to not pay due attention to what my intelligence should tell me are the bitter consequences of these actions, is to court my own disaster.

The Need to Form Conscience

It follows that I must use my intelligence to seek the truth in order to form a sound conscience and to correct an erroneous one (*VS* 61–64). That means I must take my bearings from the various sources of truth—my own perceptions, natural law, a sound education, traditional wisdom, the advice of friends, the Church, and so on.

All these aid me in coming to a correct assessment of a potential action. It also follows that my freedom is not absolute, but rather is a freedom for truth, a freedom to search out, discover, and follow the truth. We are not free to decide for ourselves what is true, to determine the truth as if it were a function of our own wills.

We cannot adopt a subjectivist deconstruction of truth in the manner of the nimble-witted Hamlet: "there is nothing either good or bad, but thinking makes it so" (act 2, scene 2). Truth is not determined by my willing it, but rather my willing something should be determined by the truth. In the grisly tradition of the will to power, Hitler, Lenin, Stalin, and Mao have shown us what happens when raw subjective will determines the truth rather than vice versa.

Conscience: Two Extremes

Two extremes seem to have emerged in the modern context. On the one hand, conscience has assumed the character of a simple subjective certainty, an absolute infallibility in the stand of the individual with regard to one or another moral issue (Ratzinger, 2). On the other hand, in the face of a profusion of authorities, conscience has tended to produce a quagmire of moral puzzlement and quandary. In an earlier age, the great Shakespeare perceived this modern perversion of "conscience," its tendency to produce moral paralysis, and immortalized it in Hamlet's famous soliloquy:

> To be or not to be—that is the question ...
> Thus conscience doth make cowards of us all;
> And thus the native hue of resolution
> Is sicklied o'er with the pale cast of thought;
> And enterprises of great pith and moment
> With this regard, their currents turn awry,
> And lose the name of action. (3.1)

Here conscience is a hindrance to action, an excess of thinking that leads to *not* doing something. Aristotle's advice had been encapsulated in the phrase *festina lente*—"make haste slowly" or better "deliberate long, act swiftly"—but here his sage advice is only half carried out.

This type of reasoning is representative of the sort of moral paralysis we often encounter today in our overblown emphasis on doubt, dilemmas, oppositions, and contrived moral "problems." Since the advent of Cartesian systematic doubt in the seventeenth century, conscience has indeed made cowards of us all.

The Nature of Conscience

But in the classical tradition conscience is far more broadly conceived and flexibly placed in relation to the virtue of prudence. Therein lies a great difference. Conscience becomes what has been called the work of prudence. As such, it has a less extreme and more moderate character. It is neither so quickly absolute, nor so paralyzingly inhibitive, as in our modern era; and the phrase "following one's conscience" conveys less of a sense of excruciating difficulty and imminent martyrdom. The truth, after all, is supposed to set us free.

What then is conscience? St. Thomas clarifies the notion in his *Summa Theologiae* under his consideration of the intellectual powers of man (I 79.13). His discussion of conscience is significantly limited to one article, indicating its partial role within the overall workings of prudence toward a moral judgment. Although "conscience" can mean a habit—the natural habit of *synderesis* (also called the "spark of conscience," the "light of conscience," or knowledge of first practical principles)—"conscience" more properly designates an act, the act of applying the knowledge of first principles to individual cases.

For "natural law discloses the objective and universal demands of the moral good, conscience is the application of the law to a particular case" (*VS* 59). Thus, synderesis is the knowledge of first principles, conscience the judgment or conclusion to which we come regarding an individual case. To put it another way, synderesis functions as the major premise of a syllogism, the particular case under consideration as the minor premise, and conscience as the conclusion.

The Formation of Conscience

Of capital importance is the fact that, as the expression of prudence, conscience in the classical tradition assumes a more flexible character. One of the parts of prudence is counsel, that is, taking counsel, which is a subordinate virtue necessary for arriving at a prudent decision. Consideration of the advice of others—or established sources of wisdom—is essential to coming to a sound moral decision, which implies that there is a social and communal dimension to the whole process of moral decision-making.

The individual must be open and not closed in on himself. No one stands alone. Rather one is born into and embedded in a community, and ideally in a coherent tradition. It should be the case that conscience is gradually formed and developed by education and experience, in the person's best interest. Thus the ignorance that leads to erroneous judgments of conscience can be averted. As we have mentioned, an erroneous conscience, which is binding and must be followed, cannot prevent one from suffering the objective effects of mistaken judgments (*VS* 63).

"No man is an island," in the realistic words of John Donne. The delusion of modern individualism is that we are all isolated individuals, who must decide for ourselves according to the light of our own consciences. This half-truth is often used to justify self-interest and the individual working his own will. But the subjective side of conscience must be complemented by the objective side. That means, "The maturity and responsibility of these judgments [of conscience] ... are not measured by the liberation of the conscience from objective truth, in favor of an alleged autonomy in personal decisions, but, on the contrary, by an insistent search for truth and by allowing oneself to be guided by that truth in one's actions" (*VS* 61).

Rev. David N. Beauregard, O.M.V., Ph.D.
Dean of Studies
Our Lady of Grace Seminary
Boston, Massachusetts

On Imposing Our Morality on Others

Pro-lifers are trying "to impose their morality" on society. So goes one of the most common one-line refutations in the bitter public debate on abortion. This is supposed to warn rational people not to be taken in by pro-life arguments, rally the pro-choice activists against a clear and present danger to decent social life and, if possible, to get pro-lifers to desist from their legislative efforts and keep their antiabortion sentiments to themselves. All this without so much as a mention that abortion kills people.

Of course, the slogan "Don't impose your morals" has great evocative power for those who prize individual freedom and the ideals of tolerant, pluralistic societies. But it also points to the deepest questions about the nature of morality and about the relation between morality and the law. Here it will be possible only to clarify some of the issues this slogan raises and to criticize its most objectionable uses.

Are Pro-Lifers Moved by Sectarianism?

The indictment against those who favor restrictive abortion laws is often based on the assumption that they are moved solely by sectarian religious convictions. Such convictions, on this assumption, should have no role in the determination of the law or public policy in modern pluralistic societies where diverse religious and non religious views about the important things in life are not only tolerated, but encouraged and cherished.

Those who favor restrictive abortion laws loudly reject this assumption. They argue soundly, in my view, that the question of who may be legally killed in a society is not a religious or sectarian question but a concern of fundamental justice, as appropriate for public debate and legal enforcement as everything else concerning a society's homicide laws. Then, they proceed to argue, on nonreligious, moral grounds, that permissive abortion laws are gravely unjust to the unborn and perhaps to others as well.

The response to this argument has been disappointing. The religious motivations of those who make it are highlighted, but the reasons they give are simply ignored. The answers to questions like the following are hardly ever considered on their merits: Is it a narrowly religious view that the unborn, as living human beings, should be consistently regarded as persons just as all other humans are? Is it only an essentially private and idiosyncratic understanding of justice which implies that, in cases of conflict between mother and child, the nod should not necessarily and always go to the mother's interests? Is it merely a religious conviction that utilitarian considerations, often disguised as public health and welfare concerns, should not justify abortion any more than they should justify other kinds of killing?

Of course, philosophers debate these matters in their journals and conferences and some philosophers answer "Yes" to all three questions. But these discussions are overwhelmed in the public debate by the repeated incantation: "Don't impose your morals on us."

Even more importantly, if the serious discussion of the questions listed above were to become better known, it would very quickly become apparent that the arguments for the affirmative answers are at least as dependent on controversial worldviews and ideologies (usually secular) as the arguments for the negative answers are dependent on traditional morality and religious belief. Is it more obvious, neutral, and objective to hold that humans are persons only if they can actually think or remember or reflect, than to hold that all human beings are persons?

Likewise, is it an unmistakable implication of justice that all recognize that maternal interests always trump fetal interests? Finally, is utilitarianism really a philosophy that is so indisputably true that its calculations should require us to abandon an ethics of killing which has stood the test of time, and which, if only utilitarianism were more strictly followed, would plainly have made the world a much happier place?

In short, the assumption that *only* those who favor restrictive abortion laws are in danger of imposing their moral views is surely false. If we are to get beyond slogans and seriously address the underlying issues about the relation of law and morality, it is by no means clear that the permissive position on abortion laws is the one we would rationally adopt.

Does Majority Agreement Make Right?

This slogan can rest on a somewhat different foundation, namely, that what is objectionable about imposing morality is that it is the attempt by a minority of people to force others to live by their moral views. Then it is the minority status of the pro-life position, not its alleged religious basis, that is being rejected.

But even assuming for the sake of the argument that the pro-life position is held by only a minority of people, this reasoning is transparently unsound. Are we to believe that might makes right? Or, more specifically, that agreement by the majority makes right and does so in such a conclusive way that even arguing in the public domain for a minority position is somehow out of line or irrelevant?

History is full of examples in which minority views, because of their power and decency, eventually become dominant. Were early abolitionists or civil rights activists committing a public sin of trying to impose their morals? If activists of former times could, and feminists, environmentalists, and other activists of today, can seek to persuade society of their viewpoints to the point of legislatively enforcing them, how can it be wrong for pro-lifers to do the same thing?

So, if there is a valid objection underlying the use of this slogan, it cannot be simply that the pro-life position is a minority view any more than it can be that pro-lifers often have religious motivations and have a viewpoint rooted in traditional morality. Is there anything deeper here? Perhaps there is.

Are the Unborn Human Persons?

For some people, the objection underlining the slogan "don't impose your morals" is that it is inappropriate to introduce restrictive legislation into such a personal area of human life. It is inappropriate because the abortion decision is so personal and affects so profoundly the intimate relationships and life prospects of those who are compelled to face it.

This objection requires a more careful response than can be developed here. Its starting point, however, is clear enough: abortion involves killing; and the killing of one person by another for whatever reason, is a serious and public matter, a concern of justice which cannot be purely private.

This initial response provokes another objection which often underlies this slogan, namely, the objection that restrictive abortion laws presuppose that the unborn are persons and, since it is not obvious that they are persons, it is unreasonable to base restrictive legislation on this presupposition.

Here again, the assumption is questionable, namely, that when the application of the concept of person is disputed, then its use is purely subjective and so should not be the basis for restrictive laws. This assumption is questionable because there are rational standards for applying the concept of person in disputed cases, in particular, the standards of simple fairness: can it be fair to exclude from personhood a class of living human beings, given that being a living human is virtually the only thing which all persons have in common?

In other words, it is arbitrary to exclude unborn humans from personhood. Indeed, it seems likely that there would be little temptation to exclude them were it not convenient to do so.

As I have already noted, the point of these preliminary responses to the serious objections which may underlie the widely employed "don't impose your morals" slogan should not be seen as anything more than a preliminary analysis. The point, rather, is that these are some of the issues which must be seriously debated if the slogan is to be anything more than an appealing bit of rhetoric which seeks to push the pro-life position aside without ever mentioning the reality that abortion kills unborn human beings. But the invitation to discuss these issues is a far cry from a one-line put-down of the pro-life effort. We in the pro-life community welcome the invitation and reject the suggestion that we have no right to speak and work for a society that respects the lives of all.

Joseph Boyle, Ph.D.
St. Michael's College
University of Toronto
Toronto, Canada

Law and Virtue

Natural Law and Human Virtue

American Culture has a curious, if not contradictory, attitude about law. On the one hand, almost all moral issues are debated as lawyerly issues. To confirm the fact that law regulates every minutia of human action, one need only peruse the Federal Register which annually runs to over 80,000 pages. Law is the medium through which debates are joined and stopped. On the eve of an important Supreme Court decision, crowds gather in front of the court like pilgrims in St. Peter's Square.

On the other hand, there is a great fear that law should ever function like law, which is to say that law should bind human choice and visit penalties or punishments on those who disobey it. As the Court opined in *Planned Parenthood* v. *Casey* (1992): "At the heart of liberty is the right to define one's own concept of existence, of meaning, of the universe, and of the mystery of human life. Beliefs about these matters could not define the attributes of personhood were they formed under compulsion of the State." Paradoxically, the chief function of law is to give citizens an immunity from virtually all positive laws.

The Flight from Legalism

This curious attitude toward law has not left the ecclesiastical culture unaffected. For the past generation, the flight from "legalism" has been a marked theme in moral theology; and yet during this same period, we have also witnessed the opposite tendency—a preoccupation with law and authority. Issues of moral theology either begin, or quickly become, issues of authority. European prelates, perhaps, will never quite understand this mindset as it affects marriage tribunals

In North America, Catholics want the law of the Church to legally dissolve one marriage and to legally validate the next one. There is scarcely a moment's thought given to the notion that law binds, and much less that the law prohibiting divorce is absolute. Instead, law is thought to be a malleable tool in the hands of an interpreting community, subserving the lifestyle goals of the parties.

Against this cultural background, we can appreciate why "virtue ethics" must be approached with a certain caution. Rather than being a focus on that part of morality which is so often neglected by an ethics of precepts, the theme of virtue can reinforce the almost neurotic preoccupation with law. Virtue ethics is liable to do so whenever it is envisaged as an alternative to, or as a substitute for, precepts which absolutely forbid some choices. If no choices are universally and absolutely wrong as to their objects, then there is no ground for those precepts which are most characteristic of law, namely, precepts which bind universally. In lieu of such precepts, the moral measure of human acts will have to be drawn either from subjective "prudence" uninformed by law, or from the *determinatio* of a positive law. Rather than providing a more balanced picture of moral phenomena, this only deepens the cycle of preoccupation and revulsion with law.

Two Principles of Human Action

St. Thomas Aquinas held that there are two distinctively different principles of human acts (ST I–II, prol. 49, 90). There are intrinsic principles such as human powers and habits. These are predicated of the nature of the person. When we speak of the excellences of the agent (his choices, the rightness of his will, his virtues, etc.) we refer to intrinsic principles of acts. However, the human act also needs extrinsic principles, among which St. Thomas mentions law and grace. An extrinsic principle is a rule and moves or governs the agent. Although a law (e.g., natural law and the new law) can be internal, in the sense of *lex inditum,* law is never intrinsic to the human agent.

In this respect, St. Thomas's distinction bespeaks the tradition common to both the classical philosophers and the theologians. The human mind is a measured-measure. It exhibits an array of perfections in the act of measuring (e.g., in prudence) only insofar as it is first measured. St. Augustine has said: "only God can be happy by his own power with no one ruling" (*De Gen. contra Mani.* II.15 §22).

The distinction between intrinsic and extrinsic principles of human acts requires that moral philosophy give proper scope to each principle. To focus on the intrinsic powers and perfections of the agent without any rule of the acts, or to conflate the rule with the powers themselves, is to imply a lawless ethics. To focus exclusively upon the extrinsic rule is to lose sight of the very thing of which moral good and evil are predicated, the agent's own choices and character. Either intrincicism or extrinsicism leads to the cycle of fascination and dread of law.

Law in Veritatis Splendor

In *Veritatis splendor* (*VS*), the Pope John Paul II tries to break this cycle. Much of the middle part of the encyclical (nn. 35–64) makes the point that there is no lawless ethics. The human person does not first possess his powers and perfections (intellect, conscience, virtue) and then have to search for a rule of his action. Man is created in such wise that he participates in a rule called the natural law. But even before the Pope engages this scholastic exercise, he tries to break the cycle of fascination and dread of law by showing the principles at work in the story of the rich young man.

The Pope notes that in the question of the young man (Mt. 19.16–21), we can see that the first and ultimate question of morality is not a lawyerly question. Unlike the Pharisees and Scribes, the young man does not ask for a legal bottom line. Morality is not merely a system of rules but rather consists of rules within a system of ends. And there is a system of ends insofar as there is an end that is truly and unconditionally worthy of our devotion. The first question concerns the good ("Teacher, what good must I do ...?). But the first response concerns the law ("if you wish to enter into life, keep the Commandments"). The Pope notes that each of the precepts "represents the absolutely essential ground in which the desire for perfection can take root and mature" (*VS* n. 17). The point of the law is the perfection of the agent, whether by the moral virtues or by the Beatitudes, which the Pope characterizes as a "self portrait" of Christ (*VS* n. 16). The moral life is not an either-or; it is not law or virtue, but both.

Consider, for example, the case of a fledgling piano player. His teacher begins, naturally enough, by teaching him the scales. Eager to exercise his own creative freedom, however, the student ignores the scalar rudiments, and instead tries to achieve the end in an undisciplined and unruled way. The teacher, of course, points out that the scales are not a merely instrumental means used for the end of making music; they constitute the inner architecture of the music. The scales are not just guidelines, nor just harmonic "stuff" out of which human liberty makes a composition. To be sure, a piano teacher who only focused upon the scales would misrepresent the activity of music. By the same token, a student who neglected the scales will never develop musical virtues.

By analogy to the moral life, human authority and freedom come into their own only if certain norms are recognized and embodied. Just as from the scales and axiomatic measures of music there can come a Beethoven sonata, or a Penderecki 12-tone composition, so too from obedience to the commandments there opens the possibility of a creative, fluid, and completely realized human liberty. The point of learning the scales is not a mindless repetition of the scales; the point is to make beautiful music. So, too, the point of the Commandments is communion with God and harmony with neighbor. There is no upper limit to our realization of these ends. But there is a foundation that is necessary and indispensable.

As Yves Simon has pointed out, a fully realized practical judgment is usually not something that can be communicated in the form of a precept (*Practical Knowledge* [New York, 1991], 24). In the sphere of art, for example, the Beethoven sonata cannot be communicated simply by imparting a rule. So, too, much of the moral life is displayed in practical judgments where the rectitude of the agent's habits (virtues) carry the day. Virtue is indeed a kind of norm. The question, however, is whether it is a *mensura prima* or a *mensura proxima.* The great tradition of moral philosophy and theology holds that virtue presupposes, even as it makes effective, antecedent law(s). There is not an autonomous virtue ethic.

Law and Virtue as Complementary

The debate between the Pope and some of the dissenting moral theologians is a debate over whether the powers and habits of a human agent are a primary rule of action. One very prominent moral theologian holds that: "Neither the Hebrew Bible nor the New Testament produces statements that are independent of culture and, thus, universal and valid for all time: nor can these statements be given by the Church or its Magisterium. Rather, it is the task of human beings—of the various persons who have been given the requisite intellectual capacity—to investigate what can and must count as a conviction about these responsibilities." On this theologians's view, the rule of action is basically the rule of reason applied to the concrete case. Law is the *ex post facto* codification of the myriad of such concrete prudential judgments. How this codification could ever decisively bind future "prudential" acts is quite mysterious.

Right here we can see the ingredients of the cycle of fascination and dread of law. For law would have to make its appearance as something over and against the adequacy of prudence operating in each concrete case. This is only a recipe for authoritarian and arbitrary use of coercion against which one feels the need to posit even greater immunity from law. And so the cycle turns.

That human order requires both the rule of law and the perfection of prudence is confirmed once we write the picture large and consider the political order. "The principle of government law," Yves Simon reminds us, "is subject to such precarious conditions that, if it were not constantly reasserted, it soon would be destroyed by the opposite and complementary principle, viz., that of adequacy to contingent, changing, and unique circumstances" (*Tradition of Natural Law* [New York, 1992], 84). Whether in the individual or in the body politic, the life of the practical intellect requires, as Simon says, two "complementary" principles: law and virtue.

Russell Hittinger, Ph.D.
Warren Professor of Catholic Studies
and Research Professor of Law
University of Tulsa
Tulsa, Oklahoma

VIRTUE OR OBLIGATION IN CATHOLIC ETHICS?

Ever since the publication of Alasdair MacIntyre's *After Virtue* (Notre Dame, 1981), virtue ethics has increasingly captured the field from those forms of ethics that center on moral rules and duties. MacIntyre has more recently argued his case in *Three Rival Versions of Moral Inquiry: Encyclopaedia, Genealogy, and Tradition* (Notre Dame, 1990), a book in which, because of its inability to resolve crucial moral differences, he dispatches the rationalist tradition stemming from the Enlightenment and the nineteenth century "genealogist" tradition stemming from Nietzsche, in favor of a return to the Aristotelian-Thomistic tradition.

Catholic Tradition and Virtue Ethics

In concert with MacIntyre's treatment of ethics on the secular scene, Fr. Servais Pinckaers, O.P., in an equally impressive book, has documented with amplitude and clarity the evolution of the Catholic tradition in moral theology. One of his main points is that, beginning in the fourteenth century with William of Occam and after the sixteenth century, virtue ethics was replaced by an "ethics of obligation" (*The Sources of Christian Ethics*, translated by Sr. Mary Thomas Noble, O.P. [Washington, D.C.: CUA Press, 1995]. Whereas during the Middle Ages the moral scheme of the Seven Deadly Sins had been generally used (see, e.g., Chaucer's "Parson's Tale"), after the Reformation and the Council of Trent, which was interested in producing sound confessors, the Decalogue became the generally accepted scheme for Christian ethics (John Bossy, "Moral Arithmetic: Seven Sins into Ten Commandments," in *Conscience and Casuistry in Early Modern Europe*, ed. Edmund Leites [Cambridge, 1988] 221).

At the end of the sixteenth century, the Gothic cathedral of virtue ethics in St. Thomas Aquinas' *Summa Theologiae* was dismantled, broken into separate treatises, and in effect replaced by the manualist tradition which concentrated on the obligations of the Ten Commandments, the laws of the Church, and specific duties. Thus, the moral universe of the Secunda Pars of the

Summa, with its constellation of the three theological and four cardinal moral virtues and their opposite vices, was reduced to a more restricted concentration on sin and law. The focus of ethics lay no longer on beatitude and the virtues but rather, in a more rationalistic and less Scriptural form, on commandments, obligations, and duties. The questions we propose to examine here are two: What are the main features of this important historical shift in emphasis, and what is its significance for bioethics?

From Virtue to Obligation

For one thing, since the end of the sixteenth century, there has been an historical loss of unity in moral theology. Gradually, speculative theology has been drawn away from the mystical, the pastoral, and ultimately the scriptural. Now directed at the administration of the sacrament of Penance and at the solution of "cases of conscience," the manuals of moral theology present a simplified fundamental morality that in reality introduces a new systematization. The treatises on law, on conscience, on human acts and on sin, form its basis, and legal obligation is its central fulcrum.

The commandments of the Decalogue and of the Church provide the divisions of "special moral," and the division between law and liberty, especially in doubtful cases, becomes the principal occupation of the moralists. The dispute on probabilism occupies all their attention and provokes their divisions with respect to the solution of cases of conscience or systems of morality. In spite of their modest intentions at the beginning, and their frequent reference to St. Thomas, the manualists inaugurate and spread a very different conception and organization of moral theology that reflects their time (Pinckaers, 254–79).

Moreover, there has been a shift in the notion of moral freedom from what Pinckaers calls a "freedom for excellence" to a "freedom of indifference." The latter emphasizes the primacy of the will in moral action, to the exclusion of natural inclinations, which are seen as threats and obstacles to free will (note that Descartes' "clear and distinct" ideas are also threatened by the obscurity caused by the disturbance of the passions). The virtues are likewise excluded because they are settled habits of acting in a certain direction that seem to reduce the liberty of the will.

Indeed, the notion of virtue itself undergoes a transformation from being understood as the perfection of a dynamic power of acting to a traditional and convenient category for systematizing moral obligations. By contrast, in a freedom for excellence, intellect is conjoined with will, and freedom is rooted in the natural inclinations and their attraction toward the true and the good, toward that which has quality and perfection. Virtue is a cultivated habit necessary to the development of freedom, and one's final end, the ultimate truth and goodness of God, is a principal element in acting freely since it unifies the various powers of the soul (Pinckaers 354–78).

Again, the two forms of freedom generate two different attitudes toward the law. The one sees law as an exterior constriction and a limitation of liberty, whereas the other views it as an external aid to the development of liberty, particularly in connection with the attraction toward the true and the good, and in the first stages of education (Pinckaers, 375).

In addition, natural law, as seen in the earlier speculative theology, is a dynamic interior law inscribed in the heart of man, drawing him by nature to God, and not an exterior limitation on his freedom. Thus he is inclined toward the good, toward the conservation of life, toward the truth, toward life in society, and he becomes free insofar as he reaches the objects of these inclinations.

Finally, and perhaps most importantly, the two forms culminate in their respective emphases on virtue and obligation, on an ethics of the virtues and an ethics of duty. The masterwork of the first tradition is St. Thomas' development of Aristotle's ethics in the Secunda Pars of the *Summa Theologiae*, with its elaborate treatment of the moral life in terms of its end, principles, passions, law, grace, and virtues; and the seminal work of the second is Kant's *Foundations of the Metaphysics of Morals,* with his famous "categorical imperatives." Elsewhere Kant defines virtue, significantly, as "the moral strength of a man's will in fulfilling his duty" *(The Metaphysics of Morals*, trans. Mary Gregor [Cambridge, 1991] 206).

Bioethics and the Virtuous Person

What is the significance of this historical shift for bioethics? Since virtue and obligation, virtue and law, are not opposed, but are complementary, bioethics must not be conceived reductively as simple rule-following, mere determination of the law, or minimal fulfillment of obligations. Rather it must be understood more fully as the virtuous activity of the whole person—doctor, nurse, or patient—in realizing the dynamic aims of nature and of God.

The determination and formulation of laws, rules, and obligations is an extremely important part of this process, but there are areas the law does not touch, e.g., the quality of care provided by medical personnel or the way in which an operation is performed. And there are fluid situations which require skill and poise beyond mere knowledge of the law. A nurse has an obligation to care for patients, but the virtuous fulfillment of this obligation in the dynamism of time takes more creative skill, intelligence, and wisdom than formulated laws and rules can provide.

Moreover, situations arise for which there are no formulated rules or laws, and in such cases the virtuous nurse or doctor can better discern what is right and good for the patient.

Bioethics, then, has need of objective laws and rules and obligations, particularly in hard or difficult cases, but it also has need of the virtues, of the subjective dispositions that enable us to act with perfection so as to bring about the good of nature and the health of the patient. Ethics involves more than a set of exterior laws and rules; it also involves the interior dispositions and perfection of the virtuous acting agent.

Rev. David N. Beauregard, O.M.V., Ph.D.
Dean of Studies
Our Lady of Grace Seminary
Boston, Massachusetts

HUMAN FREEDOM AND NATURAL LAW

Without a doubt, one of the determining causes of the present crisis in Catholic morality is the critique, if not the jettisoning, of the teaching on natural law. Associated with the Decalogue, natural law had served as a fundamental basis of the Church's traditional teaching on morality and had furnished the classical manuals with their main divisions of subject matter according to the Ten Commandments. One of the principal aims of Pope John Paul II's encyclical *Vertitatis splendor* (*VS*) is to firmly reestablish this basis, which can equally serve as the foundation for the definition and defense of human rights.

The encyclical is not content with reaffirming the validity of the natural law. It undertakes to demonstrate in quite an original way the relationship of the natural law to freedom, reason, and conscience, and to show that they exist in harmony, not opposition.

With this object the encyclical refers explicitly to the teaching of St. Thomas Aquinas, invoked by Leo XIII in one of his letters (*VS*, n. 44). The best preparation for reading the encyclical on this point is to recall the main features of the Thomistic analysis of natural law. For the Angelic Doctor natural law is, like every law, ordered by reason, but it is a law interior to man. It is a participation in the eternal divine law and serves as a foundation for civil law. It corresponds to the Decalogue within the Mosaic law and finds its fulfillment in the New Law taught by Christ in the Sermon on the Mount (ST I–II, 108). It is also found in such witnesses of the great philosophical tradition as Cicero, who inspired St. Thomas. In his *Republic* (III, 22), Cicero says:

> True law is right reason in agreement with nature; it is of universal application, unchanging and everlasting; it summons to duty by its commands, and averts from wrongdoing by its prohibitions .... And there will not be different laws at Rome and at Athens, or different laws now and in the future, but one eternal and unchangeable law will be valid for all nations and times, and there will be one master and ruler, that is, God, over us all .... Whoever is disobedient is fleeing from himself and denying his human nature, and by reason of this very fact he will suffer the worst penalties, even if he escapes what is commonly considered punishment.

Natural Law as the Light of Reason

In the first place, contrary to common opinion, natural law is not the expression of the pure will of God imposing a code of obligations and prohibitions. It is the work of the wisdom of God, imprinting his law within the human reason which He enlightens and within the human heart which He inclines to the good. Natural law is "nothing other than the light of understanding infused in us by God" (*VS*, n. 40). Thus it corresponds to the essential link which the encyclical affirms between freedom and truth, serving as the touchstone and first principle of all its reflection. Receiving this light, reason is able to show us what our nature is and where our good lies, who are the persons and what are the circumstances affected by our actions, and the moral quality of our actions. In this way we can participate actively in the divine government and discern what is good and what is evil for ourselves and for others (*VS*, n. 43).

Natural Law as Interior Inclination

The natural law does not impose itself upon us from without, as do the laws of physical nature or civil prohibitions. It affects us from within, in the form of deep inclinations which move us, in the intimacy of our hearts, toward the end destined by our spiritual nature, toward the happiness to which God calls us (*VS*, n. 43). The encyclical frequently cites the five natural inclinations noted by St. Thomas: desire for the good, the instinct of self-preservation, the generation and rearing of children, the seeking of truth, and the cultivation of social life. It adds to these the contemplation of beauty (*VS*, n. 51). The chief precepts of the natural law flow from these inclinations, as do also the fundamental human rights and duties.

We note that some of these inclinations obviously belong to the spiritual order, such as the sense of good, truth, and justice, and that others include a determining biological dimension, such as the sexual instinct. But the encyclical insists strongly, with good reason and in complete conformity with the thought of St. Thomas, on the profound unity which integrates body and soul in the human person in a "unified totality," especially when considered as a moral subject. All the natural inclinations work together in a concrete moral action. We cannot "dissociate the moral act from the bodily dimensions of its exercise" (*VS*, nn. 48–50), and this applies particularly in the case of sexual activity and the issues concerning it, where the biological and moral planes really cannot be separated.

Natural Law as Participation in God's Wisdom

The natural law is not isolated. It is part of that vast movement of activity which comes forth from the wisdom and goodness of God and returns to him. The natural law is first an emanation of the eternal law, but it takes on a special mode in man owing to his reason, which renders him capable of self-direction and free action. Subject to God as a creature, man cannot pretend to create good and evil; but he should become a collaborator with God by freely accomplishing the good which he discerns in the light of reason and conscience. Thus he enjoys a real autonomy, which can be qualified as a "participated theonomy" (*VS*, n. 41), or participation in God's governance.

Natural law has been equally enlightened by divine revelation. In the Old Testament it was included in the law of God given on Mount Sinai "as a particular gift and sign of the divine covenant." The psalms sing of this law as a source of happiness and refreshment for the soul (*VS*, n. 44). It finds its fulfillment in the New Law which St. Thomas defines as an interior law, written by the Holy Spirit in the hearts of the faithful and working through love (*VS*, n. 45).

Veritatis splendor rightly insists on the coordination of these various laws; it is useful to distinguish them for purposes of study, but they converge to throw light on things to be done like rays issuing from a single source of light. These laws cause us to participate in the design of God's wisdom and love and contribute to God's reproducing in us the image of his Son (*VS*, n. 45).

The Harmony between Freedom and Nature

Throughout this exposition the encyclical faces up to the opposition between freedom and nature posed by certain theologians. These latter view nature as purely biological or social raw material subject to the procedures of science and technology, and as included in the category of "premoral" or "physical" goods. According to them, the teaching of natural law stems from the concepts of a physicist, a biologist, or a naturalist. These theologians argue that this teaching needs to be replaced today by the acceptance of a freedom that creates its own values and understanding of behavior. Here we find ourselves in the Cartesian tradition, which separates the body, belonging to nature and animality and viewed as a mechanism, from the spirit, the source of reason and freedom.

Vertitatis splendor takes a very clear position concerning these fundamental problems, in favor of a concept which unifies and harmonizes the human person in his various elements and activities and in his relationship to nature, understood as spiritual as well as bodily. This viewpoint proceeds from a keen awareness of the primacy of the person as a free and moral subject, created in the image of God and ordered to God. It also corresponds to a major concern of John Paul II in his other encyclicals, which is to reestablish the preeminence of ethics over technology.

Rev. Servais Théodore Pinckaers, O.P.
Professor Emeritus, University of Fribourg
Fribourg, Switzerland
(Translated by Sr. Mary Thomas Noble, O. P.)

Principles of Catholic Bioethics

Christ-Centered

Christian Anthropology and Happiness

In our political tradition, the pursuit of happiness is one of the inalienable rights with which we have been endowed by our Creator. The pursuit, however, may seem doomed to failure, which is why, perhaps, in the *Salve Regina*, our lives are said to be lived in a Vale of Tears. Have we a right to pursue the unattainable? Is life, in the grim existentialist phrase, a useless passion?

The Christian understanding of happiness operates on two levels: first, a level of insight common to believers and unbelievers alike, and, second, the level specifically based on the Christian concept of happiness, which builds on but does not destroy the common human understanding. Centuries of Christian reflection on the philosophies of Plato and Aristotle have, at the first level, clarified the positions of the two great pagan thinkers and, at the second, related their thought to the specifically Christian understanding of the ultimate purpose of life.

Happiness as Ultimate End

Happiness (*eudaimonia*, *felicitas*) is the term pagan philosophers use to express the overriding aim of human free action, the ultimate end. A human act is, by definition, one undertaken for some end or purpose. If it is true that each human act is for the sake of an end, the ends are as numerous and various as the acts themselves. But the ends of some acts are ordered to the ends of other acts, and we can gather acts into clusters insofar as they share a subordinating end.

The bricklayer, glazier, plumber, and electrician each has a particular function aimed at a specific end, but they are all ordered to the goal of constructing a building. So too the artillery, cavalry, quartermaster corps, and infantry each has its end, but they are subordinate to the ultimate purpose of the army, victory. Such considerations led philosophers to ask if there is an ultimate end, not just of clusters of acts, but of all human acts. It is in the attainment of that ultimate end that human happiness consists.

That overriding human good is both one and many: the single overall aim, and the many types of action ordered to it. What insures the ordination of types of action to the good is virtue, and of course, since there is a plurality of types of act, there is a plurality of virtues. The dominant virtuous activity, according to Aristotle, is contemplation, and the object of contemplation is the divine. The arts and skills, the moral virtues, the whole panorama of the active life, are all subordinated to the contemplation in which true human happiness consists.

The Christian Vision

It is not surprising that Christians have found the above vision of human life in many ways attractive. When the Holy Father, John Paul II, sets forth the Christian conception of the point of human life in *Veritatis splendor,* he employs the Gospel story (Matt. 19:16–21) of the rich young man who asks Jesus what he must do to in order to be saved.

The moral values presented in that story are not unrelated to the idea of human good of the Greek philosophers. The rich young man is seeking that which will make sense of the whole of his life. Keep the Commandments, Jesus replies, and the young man says he has already been doing that. Then Jesus tells him in what a perfect life consists: Go sell all you have, give it to the poor and come follow me.

The Commandments to which Jesus refers are, as he makes clear, those of the Decalogue given to Moses on Mount Sinai. Are these Commandments a matter of divine revelation? Obviously yes, in the sense that God revealed them to Moses and we read of them in Scripture.

On the other hand, the proscriptions of murder, theft, adultery, and lying do not apply only to Jews or believers. Clearly God sometimes tells us things we already know or should know. That the precepts of the Decalogue are of this kind is clear from the fact that they are present in cultures uninfluenced by revelation.

The Gospel story illustrates, accordingly, how what humans can naturally know about the way we ought to act becomes part of the full Christian account of what perfection is. But this raises problems. If the philosopher speaks of happiness as a good achievable by action, the Christian knows that true happiness presupposes a gratuitous gift of God. Both terms of the contrast are frequently misunderstood. On the one hand, Aristotle's teaching has sometimes been taken to mean that happiness is wholly within our power. A Kant will even suggest that whatever lies outside our freedom is irrelevant to the ethical, much as the Stoics held that the slings and arrows of outrageous fortune cannot alter or affect the happiness of the virtuous man.

If the grace of salvation is understood as something that simply happens to us, with no voluntary action involved, the attainment of true happiness would obviously be something altogether different from the view of true happiness derived from the philosophical analysis of human action. But clearly the grace that salvation requires modifies and elevates virtuous action such that it can, thanks to grace, merit salvation.

Imperfect and Perfect Happiness

There is a further problem. If the pagan philosophers developed a different understanding of the ultimate end of life than that towards which Christians strive—the beatifying vision of God in the next life—must not these be rivals, such that if one is true the other is false? How can human beings have two *ultimate* ends?

There cannot, of course, be two ultimate ends. The relation between the natural order and the supernatural order suggests the solution. St. Thomas Aquinas regarded the philosophical account of ultimate end as imperfect, requiring completion by what has been revealed to us by Christ. Nonetheless, if Aristotle regarded his account as an adequate statement of the whole point of human life, Thomas's reconciliation of the two would be impossible. But Thomas finds in the text of Aristotle an indication that the philosopher saw his account of the purpose of life as merely the best we could do but not in every way the complete fulfillment of our desires.

This complementarity between reason and faith on the very starting point of moral inquiry—what should be our ultimate aim in acting?—means that an already alert inquirer awaits the Good News. The young man knocking on the brothel door is looking for God, Chesterton said. Augustine, in the *Confessions,* cries out, "You have made us for yourself, O God, and our hearts are restless until they rest in you."

Without the union of God attainable through the grace of Christ, a happiness totally fulfilling of human desire and which can never be lost, man would not be a useless passion, as for the existentialist. But neither would the full potential of our nature, subordinate to grace, have been reached.

Happiness and Luck

The English word "happiness" suggests "that which *happens*," and there is no doubt that luck is needed for the attainment of the imperfect happiness of the philosophers, as grace is needed for perfect happiness. Our freedom is not complete autonomy. But in the moral sense, happiness is an achievement, not something randomly bestowed. Some are luckier than others, and this affects what their responsible actions can achieve. With respect to the true ultimate end, man's perfect happiness, God wills all men to be saved; the invitation of grace is a standing one addressed to all, but it must be accepted.

The pursuit of happiness is not so much a right or a duty as a description of the human agent, how we all act by nature. Any choice is implicitly aimed at happiness, but happiness in its full sense is unattainable in this life. On this pagans and Christians, unbelievers and believers, are agreed. The remedy for the Fall has raised us to a higher calling, to be at one with God and to see even as we are seen.

Ralph McInerny, Ph.D.
Jacques Maritain Center
University of Notre Dame
Notre Dame, Indiana

Christ as Moral Example and Teacher

Before looking at Christ as moral example and teacher, let us look at what it means to be a moral example and teacher. Let us be philosophical and define our terms. But let us also be practical and ask first how important this question is.

I think it is perhaps the second most important question in the world, the second most important question anyone can ask. This is the question Plato's *Meno* begins with, the most practical of all moral questions: Can virtue be taught? How do you make people good? (Beginning with yourself, of course.) The only more important question I know is the question the Philippian jailer asked St. Paul: "What must I do to be saved?" That is the most important question in religion. How to make people good, or how virtue comes to us, is the most important question in morality.

Five Ways to Moral Goodness

In the very first paragraph of the *Meno*, Plato mentions four possible answers to the question, "How does virtue come to us; how to make people good?" These correspond to the four basic answers philosophers would give for the next 2,400 years, both in the East and in the West. Meno asks:

1) Can virtue be taught?

2) Or, if not, is it acquired by practice?

3) Or do men have it by nature?

4) Or does it come in some other way?

Plato answers "yes" to the first question; Aristotle answers "yes" to the second; Rousseau answer "yes" to the third; and Hobbes answers "yes" to the fourth, if "some other way" is taken to mean "against nature" in contrast with the previous answer, which is "by nature."

When someone who is instructed by experience and life rather than by philosophers raises this question, however, he is likely to embrace no one of these four solutions, but instead a fifth. For he knows by experience how he has in fact learned morality: by example. That is also how religion is in fact taught most effectively. The disciples of Jesus (and of Buddha, and of other religious founders) *showed forth* something that the rest of the world longed for and "bought into." "Whatever it is that these people have, we want *it*, because we want to be like *them*." The failure to teach by example is the reason why Christians are not reevangelizing Western civilization. Chesterton says: The only unanswerable argument against Christianity is Christians. The answer to "the decline of the West" can be found in any mirror.

Children learn morality—and immorality—the same way they learn religion—and irreligion: by comparing "the good guys" with "the bad guys." Since their small slice of life cannot be counted on to supply all the right examples at all the needed times, literature steps in as a kind of second life, or representative life. Children learn morality primarily through their own real life stories in their families, and then through stories that appeal to the moral imagination. Next to the family, the moral imagination is the most powerful teacher of morality.

The philosophical reason for this is obvious. The reason why every culture, including ours, has taught morality through "media" is that we are not angels. We learn through data, through experience, through example and induction. Angels begin with abstract principles, Platonic essences. We begin with Uncle Harry. That is why Jesus taught in parables, instead of philosophy. Chesterton says there are only two things we never get bored with: persons and stories. Hell wins more citizens through boredom and indifference than through rebellion. Concrete examples, in life and in stories, are not boring but are wonderfully and interestingly complex.

Popular Alternatives

Three popular alternatives to a morality of concrete characters with moral character are:

1) Legalism: a simple "obey the rules" (still popular today in practice, though not in theory).

2) Relativism, "feel your way along as you go, create your own values."

3) Abstract Formalism à la Kant: "have a good will, good intention, be sincere, and try to do the right thing" but without any concrete information about what things are the right things (that is, intrinsic goods, the things good in themselves).

Kant explicitly rejects teaching morality by example (in a long footnote in *The Metaphysics of Morals*), even the example of Christ. He argues that we must first judge examples as fitting or not by applying prior principles, and he applies this even to Christ. So we must judge Christ as coming up to our moral principles (or not!) rather than vice versa. It sounds incredibly arrogant (though this is surely not Kant's intention). The fact is we do not even judge our human teachers merely by abstract *a priori* principles, but we learn these principles first from our parents' examples rather than judging our parents by *a priori* principles.

Christ as Supreme Example

The Christian, now, is in an incredibly privileged position to learn morality because he has not only many good examples—the saints—but the supreme "example" of God himself in the flesh (see *Veritatis splendor* [*VS*] n. 2). The Kantian puzzle of whether you judge the concrete example by means of the ideal archetype or whether you learn about the ideal archetype by experience of examples is overcome by the Incarnation, in which the divine archetype and the concrete example are one. What was incarnated in this one example was the archetype itself—not a god but God; not *a* moral being but *the* ideal moral standard, perfection itself. So even if Kant were right and morality could not be taught by example because no earthly example is good enough to be beyond criticism, this difficulty would be overcome by the Incarnation.

Christ and the saints teach us morality by a kind of mutual reinforcement: on the one hand, we understand Christ through his saints, but on the other hand we also understand the saints through Christ. Without reading the Gospels and meeting Christ there, without experience of his personality, we would not understand similar personality traits when we met them in the saints—for instance, their strange blend of very tender compassion and very tough courage, their tremendous concern with and sensitivity to suffering in others and their almost fanatical unconcern with and insensitivity (as it seems) to suffering themselves.

If all I have said is true, no more catastrophic error in teaching morality could possibly be perpetrated than the neglect of direct immersion in the four Gospels and in the lives of the saints. Young people respond to heroic challenges. They are often idealistic, open, generous, and eager for adventure, even sacrifice, if only they see the beauty of the ideal. They do not see that beauty in abstract principles; they see it in concrete examples, above all in Christ himself. They are not willing to live and die for abstractions, but they are willing to live and die for persons (not for abstract "personhood" but for persons)—just as soldiers are not willing to die for an ideology or an abstraction like "democracy" or "freedom" but *for their buddies*.

Compare three different ways of teaching "responsible decision making," or how to choose what to do in different situations (what used to be called the honorable moral subscience of casuistry). First, the Bad Old Days often used a quasi-mathematical legalism in calculating how to apply unchanging principles to changing situations. Second, the new way is to feel your way in—with vague feelings rather than abstract principles. Now both principles and feelings play essential (but very different) roles in morality; but both lack the most essential thing: concrete examples. In Christ and the saints we find both principles and feelings embedded in actual concrete personalities and events.

Meeting these persons—above all Christ—is the end as well as the means to morality. We become moral by meeting Christ, and we meet and understand Christ better the more moral we are (for moral "purity of heart" is the access to "seeing God" [Matt. 5:8]). Christ is much more than moral example and teacher (both through words *and* example); he is assuredly not less. Christ teaches us what morality is, *and* morality teaches us who Christ is. Immoral people do not understand him. They may wonder what he thought he would get out of it, or wonder whether he was a masochist. Only the pure in heart see God, and only the pure in heart understand God incarnate. So we need to be moral before we can understand Christ as supremely good. But we also need the perfect example of Christ to truly teach us morality. It works both ways.

The Christ of the Gospels is the same one who as the *Logos*, "The true light, which enlightens everyone ... " (John 1:9; see *VS,* n. 2), has already been teaching us morality from within, as our "interior master" (Augustine) from our earliest days. When we meet him in the Gospels we do not meet a stranger. It is like an amateur chess player meeting the world's champion, or a surfer meeting a wave. The God-shaped hole in our heart is confronted with the missing piece, the keystone, the cornerstone. When he is let in, he reshapes into his image all the other stones of the building that is our personality. Christ teaches morality not only by word or even by example. The most important way Christ teaches morality is by his real presence.

Peter Kreeft, Ph.D.
Professor of Philosophy
Boston College
Chestnut Hill, Massachusetts

The Mystery of Suffering

The problem of suffering is the ultimate Gordian knot, the ultimate insoluble problem, that finally ends in mystery. Why do we suffer? Or, to put the question most acutely, why do the innocent suffer? No answer seems all that adequate to the question. The various traditions and schools of philosophy give us answers that bring only partial consolation. If the cause of suffering is our illusions (Hinduism), or if it springs from the disturbance of our passions (Stoicism), or if it comes from our lack of self-knowledge (the Greeks), if we suffer in punishment for our sins (Judaism), then still the question remains—why do the innocent suffer, who in one case or another are free of illusion, passion, lack of self-knowledge, and sin? Even if suffering is simply absurd (existentialism), again there is no adequate answer to the question.

King Lear and Job

Two literary works give us some important insights. In Shakespeare's *King Lear*, the Bard's most poignant representation of the problem, an aging and feeble-minded king undergoes agonizing punishment from his cruel daughters for his excessive naïveté, rash impetuousness, and uncontrollable anger, only to see his virtuous daughter, the innocent Cordelia, hanged at the end of the play. In the midst of his pain Lear cries out to his dead daughter:

> Why should a dog, a horse, a rat, have life,
> And thou no breath at all? (5.3)

Since Lear has sinned, since he has not "seen" the good and evil in human nature correctly and has not restrained his anger, he is punished for his blindness and his inability to restrain himself. Shakespeare's answer to the problem is that human evil is the source of Lear's suffering, emanating as it does from the weakness of his uncontrolled anger and from the malice of his evil daughter's cruelty. Suffering stems from sin and lack of self-knowledge, or, in Thomistic terms, from ignorance, incontinence, or malice (*Summa Theologiae,* I-II, 76–78).

The author of the *Book of Job* poses the problem in more extreme terms, since the main character is innocent and his suffering explicitly permitted by

God himself (Job 1:1, 8, 22; 2:3, 10). Unlike Lear, Job does not suffer because of his sins—one of the "givens" of the work is that he is innocent—but simply because God acts out of a whirlwind of mystery. The various counselors who try to convince him that God is just, that he must have sinned, that there must be some humanly discernible explanation for God's actions, are twice rebuked by God himself at the conclusion of the work, just as Job is twice praised for his truthfulness—"I am angry with you [Eliphaz] and with your two friends; for you have not spoken rightly concerning me, as has my servant Job" (42:7, 8). Thus, the answer to the question "Why do the innocent suffer?" is that there is no humanly discernible answer, that human beings cannot presume to explain God's ways, that all is locked up in mystery.

Partial Answers on the Natural Plane

However, from the rich deposit of religious and ethical traditional wisdom, we can discern several reasons for suffering that explain some of its roots. It may be that it arises from illusion, from the fact that we fail to see accurately certain situations. We may, for example, give our love or our money to someone in an act of trust, and experience the pain of disillusion or loss. Thus the truth of the Hindu tradition is partially validated. Or we may give way to our passions to the point of excess, and the disorder of our passions will bring us pain. Thus the pain of King Lear, who gives way to excessive anger and ends a broken man, gives support to the Stoic tradition. Or we may sin and suffer as a consequence. Witness the adultery of King David and his subsequent suffering. These are all partial answers to the problem, and they may all overlap, since illusion, passion, and sin can all be aspects of the same person's situation. The disorder of sin can encompass all three aspects.

Transformation in Christ

In the figure of Christ and in his transfiguration, we have a hint of the ultimate answer. Suffering can transform us. It can perfect us and unite us by participation in fellowship with Christ. St. Paul says "we even boast of our afflictions," and he goes on to spell out the sequence of spiritual steps that lead to hope—"knowing that affliction produces endurance, and endurance, proven character, and proven character, hope" (Rom 5:3–4). That is, suffering perfects us and in perfecting us brings us hope of salvation. He adds (2 Cor 1:5–7): "For as Christ's sufferings overflow to us, so through Christ does our encouragment also overflow.... Our hope for you is firm, for we know that as you share in the sufferings, you also share in the encouragment."

Purgation, purification, and the way to perfection indeed imply suffering, as St. John of the Cross indicates: "the soul is as powerless in this case as one who has been imprisoned in a dark dungeon ... until the spirit is humbled, softened, and purified, and grows so keen and delicate and pure that it can become one with the Spirit of God" (*Dark Night of the Soul* 2.7.3). The most trenchant modern treatment of the problem, Pope John Paul II's *Salvifici doloris* (*SD*) makes much the same point: "Suffering must serve *for conversion,* that is, *for the rebuilding of goodness* in the subject, who can recognize the divine mercy in this call to repentance" (*SD*, n. 12, my emphasis).

The Revelation of Christ

But what of instances in which there is no natural disorder, no illusion, excessive passion, or sin? Here we rise above the natural world, as it were, to the supernatural dimensions of the problem. Above all humanity, Christ is innocent, sinless, undeserving of punishment and suffering. And yet as an expression of his love for the Father and for us, his preaching of the truth leads to suffering, which he willingly accepts. Ultimately, Christ's suffering is revealed as atonement and redemption, expressing God's forgiveness and salvific love. It leads to his glorification. In the old ninth-century Anglo-Saxon poem "The Dream of the Rood," the Rood (or Cross) explains its history, which begins in disgrace as it is cut down and then brought to the place of crucifixion, where Christ embraces the Cross, which suffers with him. Beginning as a mere tree, proceeding through the disgrace of the passion and crucifixion, the Rood ends up as an object of veneration adorned with jewels at the points where Christ's hands and feet were nailed. With profound theological insight, the author then calls the Rood the "glory-tree." Just as Christ is transfigured, so the tree joined to him in suffering is finally transformed and glorified. In his ornate seventeenth century prose Sir Thomas Browne puts it rather eloquently:

> ... if any have been so happy as truly to understand Christian annihilation, ecstasies, evolution, liquefaction, transformation, the kiss of the spouse, gustation of God, and ingression into the divine shadow, they have already had an handsome anticipation of heaven; the glory of the world is surely over, and the earth is ashes unto them.
>
> *Hydriotaphia, Urn-Burial*

Suffering and Bioethics

How do we deal with suffering in a bioethical context? To be sure, medical technology can alleviate most suffering, but it has limits. "The task of medicine is to care even when it cannot cure" (*Ethical and Religious Directives*, Pt. 5, Introduction). "Patients should be kept as free of pain as possible so that they may die comfortably and with dignity, and in the place where they wish to die ... Patients experiencing suffering that cannot be alleviated should be helped to appreciate the Christian understanding of redemptive suffering" (ibid., n. 61). As Pope John Paul II says, "Human suffering evokes compassion, it also evokes respect" and it is present in the world "in order to unleash love in the human person" (*SD*, nn. 4, 29). Thus we can feel and express human compassion and loving care for those who suffer. In order to avoid the mistake of Job's friends, we must adopt the position that we are powerless to explain and cure some aspects of suffering. After a certain point, theological explanations, ethical principles, and medical procedures are of little help, and then the aforementioned virtues properly come into play. There is no substitute for the human virtues of compassion, respect, and love. The patient in a hospital bed, after all, is not looking for an explanation for his suffering; he is looking for the consolation of compassion and hope. Ultimately the only satisfactory answer to his condition is redemption, which only faith in Christ can bring him. As for us, Shakespeare makes the relevant point at the end of *King Lear:*

> The weight of this sad time we must obey;
> Speak what we feel, not what we ought to say. (11.329–30)

David N. Beauregard, O.M.V., Ph.D.
Dean of Students
Our Lady of Grace Seminary
Boston, Massachusetts

Reflective Action

Stewardship, Dominion, and Autonomy

The Church is a player on the ethical scene. Hence she uses the language of ethical discourse in her task of speaking to the men and women of every epoch in a language they can understand. It is in this light that I will begin an examination of three words often used in ethical discourse today: *stewardship, dominion*, and *autonomy*. While it is true that many contemporary movements—feminism, for one, environmentalism, for another—will utilize one or two of them (usually *autonomy* and to some lesser extent *dominion*), it is nevertheless the case that the Catholic Church remains rather unique in her employment of all three concepts to help her sons and daughters understand the moral demands of following Christ.

While all ethical discourse is relational, Catholic included, not all contemporary ethical discourse is relational in the two senses of being both horizontal and vertical. Human beings have obligations to each other and to the world around them, to be sure, and this is what we call the horizontal dimension of ethics. But we also have obligations to the God above us, and this is the vertical dimension. An ethic based on only one dimension, the horizontal ethic of secular humanism, for example, detailed so well by Dr. Pellegrino in his article above [13–16] on human compassion, will have a far different look than an ethic based on both. Our study of these three concepts involves us in nothing less than the heart of an authentic Christian anthropology: the creature is indecipherable without reference to the God who creates.

Definition of Terms

Autonomy is a word often used by philosophers, especially since the time of Kant. Thomas Shannon gives a standard definition: "Autonomy is a form of personal liberty of action in which the individual determines his or her course of action in accordance with a plan of his or her own choosing." As *Gaudium et spes* (*GS*) makes clear, when properly understood, *autonomy* is in full concordance with the Christian message:

> If by the autonomy of earthly affairs we mean that created things and societies themselves enjoy their own laws and values which

> must be gradually deciphered, put to use, and regulated by men, then it is entirely right to demand that autonomy. Such is not merely required by modern man, but harmonizes also with the will of the Creator. ...

Improperly understood, however, *autonomy* proves destructive of authentic human good:

> But if the expression ... is taken to mean that created things do not depend on God, and that man can use them without any reference to their Creator, anyone who acknowledges God will see how false such a meaning is. For without the Creator the creature would disappear (*GS,* n. 36).

Note how the Second Vatican Council brings the perennial concerns of an authentic Christian anthropology to the forefront.

Dominion is perhaps best comprehended biblically as a sharing by human beings in the creative action of God in the world. The *locus classicus* for this notion is found in the first chapter of Genesis:

> God created man in his image, in the divine image he created him; male and female he created them. God blessed them, saying: "Be fertile and multiply; fill the earth and subdue it. Have dominion over the fish of the sea, the birds of the air, and all living things that move on the earth" (Gen.1:27–28).

In a sense, the rest of the Bible is a commentary on this notion.

The Limits of Human Dominion

One of the major concerns of Christian moral reflection is to answer such questions as the following: How far does this dominion of human beings extend? How far does God wish to share his creative action with his creatures? Much of the history of contemporary moral theology is wrapped up in the answers given to these questions. While such an excursus would be fascinating, it would take us too far afield. Suffice it to say: while it is true that God shares his power and authority, his dominion, if you will, with humanity, God never ceases being God and we never cease being creatures. Especially does this Lordship of God hold true in matters of life and death, where proper human dominion must not be confused with total control:

> On a more general level, there exists in contemporary culture a certain Promethean attitude which leads people to think that they can control life and death by taking the decisions about them into their own hands (*Evangelium vitae* [*EV*], n. 15).

Such a view is unwise and unbiblical. Human life and death are thus in the hands of God, in his power: "In his hand is the life of every living thing and the breath of all mankind," exclaims Job (12:10). "The Lord brings to death and brings to life; he brings down to Sheol and raises up" (1 Sam. 2:6). He alone can say: "It is I who bring both death and life" (Deut. 32:39) (*EV*, n. 39).

Stewardship is part of the continuing commentary on the biblical concept of *dominion*. Indeed, the good steward is the person who exercises his God-given autonomy for the good not only of self, but also of the others entrusted to the care of the steward. Here too, the steward has free range of action, yet this freedom understood in the sense of *autonomy* and *dominion* is not unlimited. Stewards *are* stewards precisely because of their relationship with the Master. Note how Fathers Ashley and O'Rourke elaborate what they call the "Principle of Stewardship and Creativity":

> The gifts of multidimensional human nature and its natural environment should be used with profound respect for their intrinsic teleology. The gift of human creativity especially should be used to cultivate that nature and environment, with a care set by the limits of human beings' actual knowledge and the risks of destroying these gifts (*Healthcare Ethics,* 3d ed., 53).

If I am not mistaken, the principle elaborated by the two Dominican scholars is a roundabout way of corroborating what we have already stated, namely, that in the Christian anthropology which grounds Christian moral reflection, God never ceases to be God and we never cease being creatures. The human being is indecipherable without a reference to the God who creates and sustains and shares dominion with his sons and daughters.

Need for a Proper Hermeneutic

Whether we speak the language of *autonomy*, *dominion*, or *stewardship*, what is crucial to grasp if we want to understand Roman Catholic moral teaching about them is that each must be seen properly as an expression of Christian anthropology. What is absolutely essential to note is that the human being is always found in the proper relation to the God who creates. Hence, magisterial documents are replete not only with the references to the three concepts but also to their correct interpretation, speaking as they often do of 'the rightful autonomy of the creature' which must be distinguished from 'any kind of false autonomy' (*GS* 41), extolling 'the rightful autonomy of man' and warning of 'absolute autonomy' (cf. *Veritatis splendor* [*VS*], nn. 35–41).

One can see the three concepts in action, as it were, in the *Ethical and Religious Directives for Catholic Health Care Services* (1995), where an attentive reading reveals their presence: the American Catholic bishops speak once of *autonomy* (introduction to Part Six) and once of *dominion* (the General Introduction). *Stewardship* occurs no fewer than eight times (and once in the notes) in the almost 10,000 word text.

One paragraph of the General Introduction to the *Ethical and Religious Directives* is especially valuable for our purposes, making reference as it does to *dominion* and *stewardship* together and linking them, as we have come to expect, with God's design for humanity:

> Created in God's image and likeness, the human family shares in the dominion which Christ manifested in his healing ministry. This

> sharing involves a stewardship over all material creation (Gen. 1:26) that should neither abuse nor squander nature's resources. Through science the human race comes to understand God's wonderful work; and through technology it must conserve, protect, and perfect nature in harmony with God's purposes. Health care professionals pursue a special vocation to share in carrying forth God's life-giving and healing work.

While it is obvious that much more could be said regarding the three notions we have been investigating, perhaps one line from the Second Vatican Council comes as close as possible to saying it best of all: "Even in secular business there is no human activity which can be withdrawn from God's dominion" (*Lumen Gentium* 36).

Rev. Germain Kopaczynski, OFM Conv., Ph.D., S.T.D.
Director of Education
The National Catholic Bioethics Center
Boston, Massachusetts

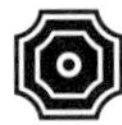

The Error of Proportionalism

What is proportionalism? Hesitant to give one formulation to the differing positions held by various theologians, Father Richard McCormick describes proportionalism in this fashion:

> Common to all so-called proportionalists ... is the insistence that causing certain disvalues (nonmoral, premoral evils such as sterilization, deception in speech, wounding and violence) in our conduct does not by that very fact make the action morally wrong, as certain traditional formulations supposed. The action becomes morally wrong when, all things considered, there is not a proportionate reason in the act justifying the disvalue. Thus, just as not every killing is murder, not every falsehood is a lie, so not every artificial intervention preventing or promoting conception in marriage is necessarily an unchaste act. (*The Tablet*, November 30, 1993.)

In large part many critics consider proportionalism to be subject to the same failings as consequentialism, and in many respects that is true. How does one calculate what are the consequences of an act? How does one measure what premoral values might outweigh the premoral evils of, say, abortion or adultery? How does one judge which circumstances justify causing premoral evils?

Proportionalism and Tradition

Proportionalists, however, claim that they are not mere consequentialists. They claim that they do not merely balance out good and bad consequences, but that they make full use of the method of moral analysis of the tradition and do so more consistently than the tradition has done. They raise questions about the consistency of the tradition in determining the object of the moral act, and how the circumstances, intention, and consequences of the action interact with the object to establish the moral evaluation of an action. Several who have responded to the rejection of proportionalism by *Veritatis splendor* have focused on these very questions.

As McCormick notes, proportionalism does consider as morally permissible some of the actions considered to be intrinsically evil by the Magisterium;

in his article he notes that proportionalism does justify acts such as sterilization, masturbation, and contraception when done for proportionately good reasons. Yet, McCormick balks at the claim of the encyclical that the principles of proportionalism justify doing morally wrong actions for a proportionately good reason. Calling the claim of the encyclical a "misrepresentation," he claims: "No proportionalist that I know would recognize himself or herself in that description."

What we have here is a classic case of "your terms or mine?" Since proportionalists do not think sterilization, masturbation, and contraception are intrinsically evil, when they justify such acts, they do not believe they are justifying morally wrong actions; they only permit premoral evil for proportionate goods. Since the Magisterium does consider such acts to be intrinsically evil, it does believe that the principles of proportionalism justify morally wrong actions. What is fundamental is that, as noted above, proportionalists admit that their principles do indeed justify what the Magisterium teaches to be intrinsically morally wrong. Why speak of misrepresentations?

The Moral Object and Circumstances

But why do proportionalists and the Magisterium disagree about the moral evaluations of such actions? It can easily seem that the source of the disagreement is that the tradition thinks some actions are intrinsically evil by their moral object and proportionalists think that no actions are intrinsically evil by their object; they are only premoral evils ("object" here means the action itself, apart from the circumstances and intention of the agent). McCormick, though, makes an interesting claim: he states: "[A]ll proportionalists would admit this [that some acts are intrinsically evil from their object] *if the object is broadly understood as including all the morally relevant circumstances.*"

McCormick fails to recognize that the tradition does indeed include all the morally relevant circumstances in the object of the act. McCormick thinks the Magisterium does this for some actions but not for others. He thinks that the Magisterium is inconsistent in allowing killing in some circumstances or for some reason (in self-defense) and not allowing sterilization in any circumstances or for no reason. This is his accusation:

> [T]he tradition has defined certain actions as morally wrong *ex objecto* because it has included in the object not simply the material happening (object in a very narrow sense) but also elements beyond it which clearly exclude any possible justification. Thus, a theft is not simply "taking another's property", but doing so "against the reasonable will of the owner". This latter addition has two characteristics in the tradition. 1) It is considered as essential to the object. 2) It excludes any possible exceptions. Why? Because if a person is in extreme difficulty and needs food, the owner is not reasonably unwilling that his food be taken. Fair

enough. Yet, when the same tradition deals with, for example, masturbation or sterilization, it adds little or nothing to the material happening and regards such a materially described act alone as constituting the object. If it were consistent, it would describe the object as "*sterilization against the good of marriage*."

This all could accept. What McCormick fails to see is that the Magisterium does define sterilization, masturbation, and contraception in the same way that it defines theft, lying, and murder. As McCormick states, "theft is taking another's property *against the reasonable will of the owner*." The "matter" of this act is "taking another's property," the morally relevant and defining circumstance is "against the reasonable will of the owner." Lying has the matter of "telling a falsehood" and the morally relevant and defining circumstance of "to one who deserves to know the truth." Murder has the matter of "killing a human being," the morally relevant and defining circumstance is that the human being is "innocent of wrongdoing deserving death."

Now consider intrinsic evils where McCormick thinks the tradition does *not* include "relevant circumstances." Sterilization (let us consider a hysterectomy) has the matter of "surgically removing one's reproductive organs" and the morally relevant and defining circumstance of "preventing conception" (which the Magisterium considers to be "against the good of marriage"). Masturbation is "the manipulation of one's sexual organs" with the morally relevant and defining circumstance of "intending to have an orgasm." Contraception is the "taking of drugs or using devices that render one incapable of conceiving" with the morally relevant and defining circumstance of preventing the sexual act from achieving its procreative end.

All actions that have the same matter could be performed under other morally defining circumstances that would make them good actions; the evils that may result would be considered to be justified by the principle of double effect. One could take what belongs to another, to save the owner's life (e.g., a gun with which the owner intends to kill himself); one can kill a human being in self-defense; one can tell a falsehood to one who does not deserve to know the truth (e.g., the Nazi searching for Jews). One could have one's reproductive organs removed for the sake of removing a cancerous growth (the prevention of conception would be the double effect); one could "manipulate one's sexual organs" for the purpose of discovering a cancerous growth (if orgasm occurred it would be the double effect); one could use drugs to regulate a menstrual cycle (the resulting infertility being the double effect).

The Magisterium is not inconsistent. Every moral act considered evil by its object has within its description some morally relevant and defining circumstances (and the intention can be considered one of the circumstances). *At this level, the real source of the debate about terminology is what counts as morally relevant and defining circumstances.* Whereas the Magisterium counts as morally defining circumstances those that transcend particular circumstances, proportionalists want to count as morally relevant and defining the circumstances of the particular agents. For proportionalists, none *of the acts described above would qualify as intrinsically evil.* For instance, if one had a proportionately good reason, given one's circumstances, to kill an innocent human being, one would be justified in doing so. The proportionalist does not think this would be an act of murder, since for the proportionalist "murder" is the "killing of an innocent human being without a proportionate reason."

For a proportionalist "killing an innocent human being" is not an intrinsic moral evil; it is a premoral evil that could be outweighed by the good consequences that the act might produce. Still, proportionalists readily admit that they think there are "virtually" intrinsically moral evils; there are acts, such as, perhaps, "killing an innocent human being" for which one can hardly conceive of a justifying circumstance. But, for the Magisterium, "killing an innocent human being" is an intrinsic moral evil called murder. It is not evil because one cannot conceive of circumstances that would justify it.

The Standard of Right Reason

The Magisterium does not accept the principle of the proportionalists, that one must weigh premoral evils to determine what is moral evil. It judges acts with their circumstances to be either in accord with right reason or not in accord with right reason. If an action is not in accord with right reason, it ought not to be done *no matter what the consequences.* The Magisterium considers sterilization, masturbation, and contraception to be against right reason, against the very meaning of the sexual act, and thus it considers them to be intrinsically evil.

So proportionalists and the Magisterium have a different standard for judging what is moral evil: proportionalists weigh and balance premoral evil and goods; the tradition speaks of acts being against right reason, against nature, against virtue (all synonymous standards, in the view of the Magisterium). What is not clear is the standard by which proportionalists judge something to be "premoral evil." They generally reject "nature" as a standard. But once they do so, it is difficult to determine what is the standard for "premoral evil." Why should homosexuality, for instance, be considered evil at all, if the sexual powers do not have a specific natural ordination? But let that question rest.

The Issue of Sexuality

What needs to be noted is the centrality of the concern with sexual ethics, central not so much to the Magisterium, but to proportionalists. Indeed, as *McCormick acknowledges, it is primarily the Magisterium's teaching about sexual matters that proportionalists resist.* Proportionalism really began with the dissent against *Humanae vitae*. It does not seem unreasonable to speculate that had *Humanae vitae* not been issued, proportionalism would not have gained the prominence it has among Catholic theologians. The Catholic tradition has unfailingly asserted that there are intrinsic moral wrongs and this has been uncontroverted until recent decades. Proportionalism followed on the heels of situation ethics and can be seen as an attempt to gain the flexibility of situation ethics while retaining the traditional terms of Catholic moral theology. Yet, situation ethics is completely incompatible with the Catholic tradition and would not have found a home there had it not served the important role of justifying the rejection of contraception as an intrinsically evil action. The Catholic tradition has always accepted that there are intrinsic moral evils; McCormick's attempt to claim that proportionalists have never denied this demonstrates that he too wishes to be part of that tradition.

It is time to spend less time on the meaning of technical terms, though it must be acknowledged that the debate spawned by proportionalists has aided in the clarification of those terms. That clarification has been made and there is no quarter on that level for dissent. What dissenters need to do is to address the Church's understanding of the meaning and purpose of sexuality, for *that* is the true source of their disagreement with the Church. It is time to have a discussion on what the goods of marriage are and how contraception, for instance, affects those goods. Such a discussion should stay as far as possible from the terms "object," "circumstances," "consequences," and "premoral evil" and speak of "personalism" and "self-mastery" and "self-giving" and of the importance of children and fidelity and heterosexuality. Pope John Paul II has provided an incredible wealth of material on these subjects. The debate on proportionalism has had its day; let us get down to the real focal point of the debate; what is sexuality for and what modes of sexual conduct are compatible with the purpose of sexuality? It is time that proportionalists faced this issue and the challenge that Pope John Paul II has given them.

Janet E. Smith, Ph.D.
Department of Philosophy
University of Dallas
Irving, Texas

Intention and the Object of Choice

Traditional Catholic moral doctrine, as formulated by St. Thomas Aquinas and recently reaffirmed in the *Catechism of the Catholic Church* (*CCC*) and in the encyclical *Veritatis splendor* (*VS*), teaches that there are three elements of a moral act which together determine the goodness or badness of that act. These "sources of morality" are 1) the object chosen; 2) the end intended; and 3) the circumstances surrounding the act (*CCC*, n. 1750, *VS*, n. 74). My purpose is to clarify these elements, especially the chosen object and the intended end, in order to make clear that acting with a good intention is not enough to guarantee the goodness of one's actions.

In simple terms, we can describe the object of a moral act as *what* a person chooses to do. The intended end is *why* the person chooses to do it. These two elements are found in every deliberate human action: a person buys medicine to regain his health; he tells a lie in order to receive a promotion; he contributes to his *alma mater* to help it carry out its educational mission. Circumstances are all those factors which make an action better or worse but do not give the act its basic goodness or badness (*CCC*, n. 1754). For example, the telling of the lie—already a bad act—becomes worse when the person injured by the lie is one's friend. Here the fact that the injured party is a friend is a circumstance. Since the fundamental moral quality of an action is determined by its chosen object and its intended end, we will focus our attention on these two elements.

Chosen Object and Intended End

The act's object is that which the agent chooses to do. Hence, the chosen object is always some action (mental or bodily). While we may at times speak of choosing a kind of food or a car or a job, we are actually choosing *to eat* this kind of food, *to buy* this car, *to carry out* this job. Even those in authority who choose what their underlings will do are choosing to command them to do those things. So, when we speak of the object of the act, we mean *that behavior which one chooses to perform*: "The object of the act of willing is in fact a freely chosen kind of behavior" (*VS*, n. 78).

It is important to avoid identifying the behavior which constitutes the act's object with the mere physical performance that the chosen behavior involves; the chosen object includes the physical behavior but is not reduced to it. For example, very different chosen objects such as the paying of a debt, a purchase, almsgiving, or bribery may include the very same physical performance: one man hands another man money. So too, the same physical performance which is sexual intercourse may be the marital act or may be adultery. A person does not choose simply to hand over money or simply to engage in sexual intercourse, but rather chooses to pay a debt or to give alms, to engage in the marital act or to commit adultery. When we speak of the act's object, then, we mean that which the person chooses to do, and not simply some physical performance.

But human action consists of some behavior chosen *for a reason.* This "reason" is the intended end; it is the "why" for the sake of which the "what" is chosen. This intended end often consists of many subordinated ends, all willed for the sake of some ultimate end. A woman buys a ticket in order to take a plane in order to be able to care for her ailing mother. In the buying of the ticket all the further ends are intended. The most important of these intended ends is the last or ultimate end, that for the sake of which all the others are willed.

Traditionally, a distinction has been drawn between the willing directed to the performance of the behavior—this willing is called "choice"— and the act of the will directed to the end for which that behavior is chosen: called "intention." These are, however, only two aspects of what is in reality a single act of willing. We distinguish them from one another because it is usually possible for a particular chosen object to be willed for different intended ends. A classic example is that of almsgiving. It is possible for a person to choose to give alms to the poor (the act's object) for the ultimate end of pleasing God (charity), but it is also possible to give alms for the end of impressing others (vanity).

Promoting the Human Good

What is it that makes a chosen object to be good or bad (or, at times, indifferent)? Those acts which promote the good of human persons are good; those which detract from that good are bad. Whether or not a given act promotes or detracts from the good of persons depends upon the structure of human nature, which in turn is part of the larger order created by God. An act such as almsgiving is intrinsically good because, by its essential structure, it promotes human welfare, while an act like adultery is necessarily evil because it directly harms the human goods of spousal love and the order of justice. So too an act such as blasphemy is in and of itself evil (*per se malum*) because it directly impedes the objective goal of human life, union with God. Some acts, such as going for a walk, are in themselves indifferent because in and of themselves they imply neither promotion nor detriment of the good. While an agent may choose to commit a given act, he does not choose whether that act accords with the created natural order or not. Rather, it is the objective order created by God which determines whether a specific kind of act is good or bad or simply indifferent. This created moral order is spelled out in the moral law, both natural and divine, which teaches us which acts are good and which bad.

Turning now to the intended end, we can say that a person's (ultimate) end is good when he intends the honest good (*bonum honestum*), that is, when he sincerely wants what is right. This good, in the Christian context, is specified as the love of God (charity), for the true ultimate end of all rational creatures is to be united by love with God. Other persons are also to be loved and their good sought, although they should be loved for God's sake and as being themselves ordered to union with God. Acts not done for this end are, in one way or another, done out of an inordinate love of self, and so we sum up the evil ends (vanity, greed, lust, power, etc.) under the rubric of self-love (*amor sui*). Whether or not a person directs his acts (and so himself) to the proper end lies with his own will; hence this ordering to the ultimate end is the most "subjective" part of the moral act, insofar as it depends wholly on the willing subject (*CCC*, n. 1752). Nevertheless, even here the agent does not determine what the proper end is, but only whether or not he will direct himself to it.

The Whole Moral Action Must Be Good

According to the traditional Catholic view, for an action as a whole to be good, *all* the elements must be good (or at least indifferent); if any one element is bad the act as a whole is bad (*CCC*, nn. 1755, 1760). That is to say, the goodness of the act arises from the integrity of all the elements (*ex integra causa*). Hence, if a person gives alms out of vanity, that person's act is evil because the intended end, vanity, is evil. The basic principle at work here is that the will is evil precisely when it wills what is evil. Similarly, the will is bad when a person wills a bad object for a good end, as occurs when terrorists bomb innocent persons for the sake of freeing their country from an unjust regime. Here, willing the murder of the innocents makes the will evil. The *ex integra causa* principle means, in short, that neither a good chosen object nor a good end alone makes a whole moral action to be good.

Let us now look at the various possible combinations of objects and ends in order to see the moral goodness or evil that they produce. In the first place, it is quite evident that when a person chooses a good object for a good end, the whole action is morally good. Equally obvious is the fact that the choice of a bad object for a bad end results in an action that is morally evil. A doctor, for example, who performs unnecessary surgery only for the end of making more money commits an evil act. More complex are those cases in which one element is good while the other is bad. If the chosen object (considered simply on its own) is good, but the person acts for a bad end, then the action as a whole is evil. Such is the case, as we have seen, with giving alms for the sake of vanity. This would be the case as well if, for example, a doctor were to perform genuinely needed procedures—good chosen objects—but did so merely out of greed. Such actions, *as performed by this person*, would be an evil.

At this point we should note a certain unavoidable subtlety that arises precisely because the chosen object and the intended end are not identical (although united in a single act of willing). If one were to ask of the greedy doctor whose doctoring really helps his patient whether or not his action was good, the answer would not be simple. If the question were directed *only* to the chosen behavior (the chosen object), then we would say that the action was good, for it truly promotes the human good. But if the question were directed to the act as a whole, including both object and end, then we must say that the action was evil. We should not think an action good just because the chosen object is good.

Euthanasia and In Vitro Fertilization

It should now be clear that any complete moral act is evil when the intended end is evil, regardless of whether the chosen act is good, bad, or indifferent. One might be tempted to infer from this that the opposite is likewise true, that whenever the intended end is good, the act as a whole is also good. But this is not so. As we have seen, bombing innocents to obtain legitimate freedom is not a good act, although the end is good. Similar instances are to be found in medicine, euthanasia being a clear case. In this instance a doctor might well be acting for a good end: to reduce the suffering of the patient.

But if the doctor chooses to kill the patient (e.g., by some lethal injection), then his action is evil because the chosen object, the killing of the patient, is evil. Despite the good intended end, the action as a whole remains evil. Less clear, perhaps, but sharing the same structure would be the case of *in vitro* fertilization. A married couple may be unable to conceive a child any other way. Now to help them conceive a child is certainly a good intended end, and there are many procedures a doctor could perform for the sake of this end and in doing so act morally well. But, as the Church teaches, the procedure of *in vitro* fertilization is not a legitimate or good means to the end of having children (*CCC*, n. 2377; *Donum vitae* II, 5). Such a procedure does not accord with the divine plan for human beings; ultimately it does not promote the good of human persons. Thus, if a doctor chooses the procedure, even for the good end of assisting a couple to conceive a child, he performs a morally bad act.

Good Intentions Are Not Enough

In short, simply to have a good intended end does not guarantee the goodness of a moral action. A good intention does not justify any and all choices. Rather, the goodness or badness of the chosen action has to be examined on its own, in the circumstances in which it is carried out, to see whether or not it is suitable. As the Church has always taught, and vigorously reaffirmed in *Veritatis splendor* (nn. 79–83), there are certain actions which are in and of themselves evil (*per se malum*) such that anytime they are chosen, whatever the intended end, the result is a morally evil act.

> If acts are intrinsically evil, a good intention or particular circumstances can diminish their evil, but they cannot remove it. They remain 'irremediably' evil acts; *per se* and in themselves they are not capable of being ordered to God and to the good of the person. (*VS*, n. 81; cf. *CCC*, nn. 1755–56).

Among the acts included in this category are procured abortion, sterilization, euthanasia, and *in vitro* fertilization. It is incumbent upon all moral agents, including health care professionals, to take the steps necessary for ensuring that their proposed chosen acts are in accord with the objective moral order. To this end they should form their consciences well by means of a thorough knowledge of the Church's teachings concerning the moral law, by appropriate consultations with other well-formed professionals, and by developing the virtue of prudence.

David M. Gallagher, Ph.D.
Assistant Professor of Philosophy
The Catholic University of America
Washington, D.C.

The Principled Decision

The Principle of Double Effect

The moral permissibility of an act which has both good and bad effects has for centuries been determined by the principle of the double effect. In recent times the principle has received much criticism from various quarters. It has been argued, for instance, that the principle is a product of the historical tradition of case comparison and that "the conditions of the principle itself have no necessary, *a priori* internal coherence" (J.F. Keenan, S.J., "The Function of the Principle of Double Effect," *Theological Studies* 54. 2 [1993], 298). The principle has also been criticized for its reliance upon intentionality and for its use as a "loophole" for justifying certain actions. What these criticisms fail to recognize is that the principle has a sound anthropological and metaphysical foundation, in particular in the three moral determinants of a good act, namely object, intention, and circumstances.

Foundation of the Principle

Aristotle began his great work the *Nicomachean Ethics* (hereafter *NE*) with this foundational truth about human action: "Every art and every inquiry, and similarly every action and pursuit, is thought to aim at some good; and for this reason the good has rightly been declared to be that at which all things aim." Aristotle recognized that every human act is performed to fulfill, complete, or perfect a person in some sense, great or small. This gives an act the character of being "good" in the sense of being something suitable, preferable, or fulfilling. One is thought to be better off, if even for a moment, than if the action were not initiated. In any event, that every human act seeks or aims at some good presupposes two important points for an understanding of the principle of the double effect.

First, if actions are undertaken precisely because the ends sought are known to be suitable and preferable, then the human being must possess something which is capable of being satisfied and completed by those ends, namely, a nature the fulfillment of which is the standard for what is *truly* good. Second, the specification of the act's nature comes from something extrinsic to the act itself, i.e., it comes from the object of the act. This is what provides the formal content of the "doing" of the action (see *Veritatis splendor,* n. 78, and *Catechism of the Catholic Church*, n. 1751). For example, acts of charity are specified as such by the good achieved for another, which is the object specifying such acts.

St. Thomas Aquinas shows that Aristotle's truth about human action is the basis for practical reason in man. The activity of reason in the area of action is itself structured and specified by whatever is thought to be good. Aquinas writes: "the first principle in the practical reason is one founded on the notion of good, namely, that the good is what all desire" (ST I-II, 94.2). It follows, Aquinas argues, that practical reason naturally apprehends man's goods as objects of pursuit and their contraries as objects of avoidance. Moreover, consistent with the metaphysical nature of action, Aquinas shows that practical reason knows what specific kinds of actions are good for man based upon the ends of natural human inclinations (see above, Servais Pinckaers, "Human Freedom and the Natural Law," 41–43).

Yet it is often the case that pursuing what is good and avoiding what is evil is hindered by the circumstances of our actions. Aristotle's *Ethics* is again the *locus classicus* for the recognition of the role of circumstances in the determination of an act's goodness. For example, in the context of discussing the difference between voluntary and involuntary actions, Aristotle describes how the pursuit of what is good can have bad effects:

> Something of the sort happens also with regard to the throwing of goods overboard in a storm: for in the abstract no one throws goods away voluntarily, but on condition of its securing the safety of himself and his crew any sensible man does so.... It is difficult sometimes to determine what should be chosen at what cost, and what should be endured in return for what gain (*NE*, 3.1).

Aristotle also recognized that the intention or reason why a person acts also affects the goodness of the act. He tells us that for an act to be virtuous it must be chosen and chosen for its own sake, i.e., it must be done with the right motive (*NE*, 2.4).

The Integrity of Goodness

Every truly good human act, then, possesses a "moral integration" of object, circumstances, and intention which constitute the integrity of goodness (see above, David Gallagher, "Intention and the Object of Choice," 73–77). This integrity consists in the concurrence of a good object, a right intention, and what Aquinas calls circumstances in due measure to the act itself (see ST I-II, 7). The claim of this article is that the integrity of the good human act, arising from the fundamental structures of human nature and action, is what the principle of the double effect is designed to protect and preserve. Based upon its protecting and preserving function, the principle's constituent parts naturally correspond to the integral components of the good human act. The fact that every human act contains the three elements of object, intention, and circumstances to which the structure of the principle of the double effect corresponds is what makes it such a useful and practical tool in the prudential judgment of cases.

The Principle Itself

The five conditions of the principle itself (some reduce them to four) may now be aligned with the three moral determinants of the human act. An act with both good and bad effects is permissible if:

With respect to the *object* of the act:

1) the act is in itself good or at least morally indifferent.

With respect to the *intention* of the act:

2) the good effect is directly intended and the bad effect is foreseen but unintended.

With respect to the *due measure of the circumstances* touching upon the effects and the act itself:

3) the good effect is not achieved by means of the bad effect;

4) the good effect is proportionate to the bad effect; and

5) the good effect can only be achieved concomitant with, but not by means of, the bad effect.

The structure of the principle necessarily aligns a moral judgment with the structure of the good act. However, structural alignment is not sufficient by itself. The structure of the principle requires that the appropriate virtues, including prudence, be brought to bear in the application of the principle to concrete cases. Let us see how the principle of the double effect is applied in a typical case.

Application to a Case

The case is that of a woman who is pregnant with a baby of sixteen weeks gestation and who is experiencing severe chorioamnionitis (infection of the chorionic and amniotic membranes). Despite treatment, the disease has progressed to the point of placing the lives of mother and child in jeopardy. The baby is at a previable stage and will not survive outside the womb. Abortion is not a moral option. The ethical question then becomes whether the act of inducing labor early is morally permissible.

The act in this case is the induced expulsion of the infected chorionic and amniotic membranes along with the (foreseen but unintended) expulsion of the fetus from the uterus of the woman. This is a good kind of thing to do. The object of this act is the preservation of life, and so the first condition of the principle of double effect, under the heading of "Object" above, is satisfied. However, the act of inducing labor would have both good effects and bad effects. The good effects of the act are the amelioration or cure of the pathology, thus saving the life of the mother; the saving of the life of the child from a certainly, or imminently threatening, lethal environment; and the allowing of an opportunity for baptism. The primary bad effects would be the early delivery and the certain death of the nonviable baby.

In order for the act to retain its goodness amidst these good and bad effects, the other four conditions of the principle must be met. The intention of the physician and mother must be treatment of the pathology, thus satisfying the requirements for a good intention (condition no. 2). The good effect cannot be obtained by means of the bad effect—the death of the child cannot be the means by which the mother's life is conserved (condition no. 3). The good effect of conserving the lives of both mother and child (to the extent possible) is proportionate to the bad effect (condition no. 4). The third condition is assured only if there is no other reliable way to secure the good effect, although it is secured concomitant with (but not by means of) the unintended bad effect of a certain death for the child (condition no. 5). Fulfillment of these last three conditions of the principle of double effect achieves a due measure of circumstances (see *Ethical and Religious Directives for Catholic Health Services* [1995], n. 47).

The use of the principle of the double effect in such a case, especially by someone who possesses the virtue of prudence, is extremely helpful towards ensuring a sound moral judgment. Contrary to what its critics claim, the use of the principle need not lapse into a legalism so long as its anthropological and metaphysical grounding in human nature and human action is taken into account. But this is precisely what the prudent person does.

Peter J. Cataldo, Ph.D.
Director of Research
The National Catholic Bioethics Center
Boston, Massachusetts

The Totality and Integrity of the Body

Man's dignity is derived from his having been created by God, and the way in which He created man is as body and soul. As Pope John Paul II teaches in his encyclical on moral theology, *Veritatis splendor* (*VS*), "The person, including the body, is completely entrusted to himself, and it is in the unity of body and soul that the person is the subject of his own moral acts" (no. 48). Man in his entirety is of a dignity far surpassing any other creature on earth. In the encyclical the Pope speaks of "the singular dignity of the human person, 'the only creature that God has wanted for its own sake' (*Gaudium et spes* [*GS*], no. 24)" (*VS*, n. 13).

This creature known as man is, to use the Pope's words, "a rational body." "Only in reference to the human person in his 'unified totality,' that is, as 'a soul which expresses itself in a body and a body informed by an immortal spirit,' can the specifically human meaning of the body be grasped" (n. 50). Hence man must be respected in his body as in his soul, in the integrated totality of his spiritual/bodily being. It is from these truths about man that the moral principles of integrity and totality are derived and applied to questions of medical morality.

Complementary Principles

The principles of totality and integrity are complementary and refer to the way in which we treat the whole person by respecting his bodily integrity and the natural hierarchy of life functions. In his *Summa Theologiae*, St. Thomas articulated the obvious truth that each member of the human body "exists for the sake of the whole as the imperfect for the sake of the perfect. Hence a member of the human body is to be disposed of according as it may profit the whole .... If ... a member is healthy and continuing in its natural state, it cannot be cut off to the detriment of the whole" (ST II-II, 65.1). In other words, an act of mutilation, the "cutting off" of a member of the body, would do violence to the integrity and totality of man as God has created him.

Usually the principle of totality is seen as directed toward the preservation of the physical whole of the human body while the principle of integrity refers to the respecting of the hierarchical ordering of the members of the body with "the values of intellect, will, conscience, and fraternity (being) preeminent" (*GS,* n. 61). As Pope Pius XII pointed out in his address to the Congress of Psychotherapy and Clinical Psychology on April 15, 1953, "Man is an ordered unit, one whole, a microcosm, after the fashion of a State whose charter, determined by the end of the whole, subordinates to this end the activity of the parts in the right order of their value and function." Because man is entirely good, in his lower bodily functions as well as in his higher spiritual activities, he may never be directly violated at any level of his being.

However, there can occur situations in which it would appear that one must sacrifice a part of the body, such as the appendix, or a limb, such as a leg, in order to preserve the life of the individual. If the person is suffering acute appendicitis, the appendix must be removed to save his life. If the individual has a gangrenous leg, he may need to have it amputated in order to avoid death. As Ashley and O'Rourke put it, "Lower functions are never sacrificed except for the better functioning of the whole person and even then with an effort to compensate for this sacrifice" *(Ethics of Health Care* [1994], 45). And *The Ethical and Religious Directives for Catholic Health Care Services* [1995] teaches that "All persons served by Catholic health care have the right and duty to protect and preserve their bodily and functional integrity. The functional integrity of the person may be sacrificed to maintain the health or life of the person when no other morally permissible means is available" (n. 29).

What Can Be Sacrificed to Save Life?

Basic human capacities cannot be sacrificed unless the person's very life is placed in danger. For example, it is possible that a man has cancer and that the hormones produced by his healthy testicles are helping the cancer to grow. Normally one may never be directly deprived of his reproductive capacities. But in this case, if he were not he could well die. Therefore, it would be legitimate to remove the testicles in order to reduce the spread of the cancer.

In 1953 Pope Pius XII taught that there were three circumstances in which one could surgically remove an otherwise healthy organ: 1) when the preservation of the organ would cause serious damage or even endanger the life of the entire organism; 2) when the damage could not be avoided in any other way than through surgery, and there is reasonable hope of success; and 3) when the surgery and removal of the organ or suppression of its function will lead to a diminution or elimination of the threat to the organism (*Acta Apostolicae Sedis*, 45 [1953], n. 14, 674).

However, this principle could not be applied to a woman who wanted to have a tubal ligation in order to avoid a future pregnancy which might prove dangerous to her health. The reason for this is that the present "nonpregnant" condition of the woman poses no health threat to her and therefore could not justify the mutilation of the body. Also, a pregnancy would result from an act of sexual intercourse in which the woman would freely choose to engage. In other words, it is a condition which she could avoid through a free act of the will.

However, it would seem to be permissible for a physician to remove a severely damaged uterus after a number of pregnancies if it was considered to be in a pathological condition which constituted here and now a danger to the woman (see Congregation for the Doctrine of the Faith, "Responses on Uterine Isolation and Related Matters," in *Origins* 24.12 [September 1, 1994], 211–212). Here the principle of double effect would be applied, i.e., an unintended evil side effect (sterility) would result from a directly willed and executed good act, the removal of a pathological uterus. In such cases, care must be exercised to be certain that one is not removing the uterus for contraceptive purposes, which would be immoral.

The *Ethical and Religious Directives* state this teaching concisely: "Direct sterilization of either men or women, whether permanent or temporary, is not permitted in a Catholic health care institution. Procedures that induce sterility are permitted when their direct effect is the cure or alleviation of a present pathology and a simpler treatment is not available" (n. 53).

Physical Integrity and Functional Integrity

The application of the principles of totality and integrity are not quite so clear when it is a question of an individual giving up part of his body to help another. The principle of totality does not refer simply to the anatomical wholeness or physical integrity of the body. If that were the case, it would be violated whenever one had a haircut or a manicure. Rather, the bodily wholeness which may not be violated is a functional one. We may do nothing which would diminish or threaten the functional integrity of the body. Consequently there is no problem giving blood for someone else who is in need of it as the result of an accident or surgery or illness.

However, it might be that a living person would want to donate an organ to a family member or friend who is in need. There is, of course, no moral problem with a living person "willing" the donation of his organs upon his death. But to provide an organ while one is still alive would seem to violate the principle of totality. This is not necessarily the case. It might be possible to donate some bone marrow for a transplant without hurting one's own body. Also, some organs come in pairs, so that the loss of one would not significantly impair the overall functioning of the body. For example, it would be possible for a living person to donate one of his kidneys to another person without being deprived of the necessary functions of the remaining kidney. However, a person would still put himself at some risk by donating a kidney. There are always risks accompanying surgery, and there would be the possibility that damage could be done to the other kidney sometime in the future. Consequently there must be a very grave reason for making such a donation.

On the other hand, one could not donate an organ such as an eye, for example, because even though eyes come in pairs, the elimination of one of them would severely diminish the wholesome functioning of the body. A person loses considerable peripheral vision and depth perception with the loss of an eye.

The *Ethical and Religious Directives* also speak to the morality of such donations. "The transplantation of organs from living donors is morally permissible when such a donation will not sacrifice or seriously impair any essential bodily function and the anticipated benefit to the recipient is proportionate to the harm done to the donor" and thc donor has given free and informed consent (no. 30).

In the Image of God

Catholic morality is based upon a profound respect for man, "the only creature wanted by God for its own sake." It is also based upon a profound respect for the body: "The human body shares in the dignity of the 'image of God' ... and it is the whole human person that is intended to become, in the body of Christ, a temple of the Spirit" (*Catechism of the Catholic Church,* n. 364). The principles of totality and integrity guide our actions in the care of this spiritual and bodily creature for whom God has such love.

John M. Haas, Ph.D., S.T.L.
President
The National Catholic Bioethics Center
Boston, Massachusetts

Ordinary versus Extraordinary Means

In 1595, at the end of the High Renaissance, the Dominican theologian Domingo Bañez made a distinction that has become classic in medical ethics: the distinction between ordinary and extraordinary means. In commenting on St. Thomas Aquinas' in his *Summa Theologiae* regarding mutilation (II-II, 65.1), Bañez asks whether one is obligated to undergo an amputation of a limb (anesthesia was unavailable in the sixteenth century). He first clearly states that ordinary means of preserving life and conserving health are morally obligatory because of the responsible stewardship humans are charged with by God. He continues:

> [A]lthough a man is held to conserve his own life, he is not bound to extraordinary means but to common food and clothing, to common medicines, to a certain common and ordinary pain: not, however, to a certain extraordinary and horrible pain, nor to expenses which are extraordinary in proportion to the status of this man... [A]lthough that means [amputation] is proportioned according to right reason and from the consequence is licit, it is, however, extraordinary. (Cited by Daniel Cronin, *Conserving Human Life* Braintree, MA: Pope John Center (1989), 42.)

The terms of the question would change with the introduction of anesthesia and antisepsis. At the beginning of the twentieth century, the question was again asked by theologians whether an amputation would be extraordinary means. This time, another nuance was added to the answer: all moralists agreed that because of more effective pain control, amputation was no longer considered extraordinary.

Also, the deprivation of physical integrity could be compensated for in some measure by the attachment of artificial limbs. While concurring with this opinion, Fr. Augustinus Lehmkuhl, S.J., makes the further distinction between pain and horror, and maintains that one need not be bound to undergo an operation that one views with a great deal of repulsion, even though, from a purely medical perspective, the course of treatment would be considered ordinary means.

The Distinction as Medical or Moral

It is important to note the significance of this theological development. There is now understood to be a difference in the way the line is drawn between ordinary and extraordinary means by medical science on the one hand, and moral theology on the other. In medicine, a means is ordinary which is 1) scientifically established; 2) statistically successful; and 3) reasonably available. If any of these conditions is lacking, the means is considered to be extraordinary.

In moral theology, a means is ordinary if it is beneficial, useful, and not unreasonably burdensome (physically or psychologically) to the patient. There is a consideration of reasonable cost as well. From the beginning of this century, with the widespread use of anesthesia and other forms of pain and infection control, the moral significance of physical pain has diminished and the psychological state of the patient (horror and repulsion) has been given more consideration.

Pope Pius XII gave magisterial expression to the distinction between ordinary and extraordinary means in his November 24, 1957, address to Catholic physicians and anesthesiologists:

> Normally one is held to use only ordinary means—according to the circumstances of persons, places, times and culture—that is to say, means that do not involve any grave burden for oneself or another. A stricter obligation would be too burdensome for most people and would render the attainment of the higher, more important good too difficult. Life, health, all temporal activities are in fact subordinated to spiritual ends. On the other hand, one is not forbidden to take more than the strictly necessary steps to preserve life and health, as long as one does not fail in some more serious duty.

In these four sentences, the Holy Father has summarized and ratified the theological tradition regarding the distinction between ordinary and extraordinary means. He does not embrace the "clinical" definition of ordinary means as entirely normative for ethical evaluation. Rather, the Pope understands the distinction to be determined by the relevant circumstances of the case in its clinical and personal dimensions ("persons, places, times and culture").

He further notes that, while one can forgo extraordinary means to begin with, one may also cease such lifesaving attempts once the means (already initiated) are determined to be extraordinary. That is, there is no moral difference between withholding extraordinary means to begin with and withdrawing them once begun. Finally, "even when it causes the arrest of circulation, the interruption of attempts at resuscitation is never more than an indirect cause of the cessation of life, and one must apply in this case the principle of double effect."

The Common Determinants

In light of the theological tradition and the Magisterium, then, the common elements employed by theologians to determine whether something constitutes ordinary means in a given case are: hope of benefit, "common use" (that is, not experimental or exotic), "according to one's status" (financially and psychologically), not difficult to use, and not otherwise unreasonable. The Church further teaches that while extraordinary means are not usually unethical to undergo, it is not morally obligatory that one undergo them (unless one is not reconciled with God or if the lives of others depend on the life of the patient).

On May 5, 1980, the Sacred Congregation for the Doctrine of the Faith issued its *Declaration on Euthanasia*. While its main teaching is about the evil of euthanasia, there is a reaffirmation of the traditional distinction between ordinary and extraordinary means, and a modification is introduced:

> In the past, moralists replied that one is never obliged to use 'extraordinary' means. This reply, which as a principle still holds good, is perhaps less clear today, by reason of the imprecision of the term and the rapid progress made in the treatment of sickness. Thus some people prefer to speak of 'proportionate' and 'disproportionate' means.

This is not to be understood as the "proportionalism" rejected by Pope John Paul II in *Veritatis splendor.* Rather, I think the Sacred Congregation recognized that there are two contrasting understandings of the distinction (medical and moral), and wished to acknowledge that the moral distinction is best understood in the language of proportion—in the sense that "proportionate" is a term used in common parlance to mean "reasonable—all things considered."

Some Examples

The distinction between ordinary and extraordinary (proportionate/disproportionate) means is applied throughout the entire range of treatment options: in arenas of non-life-threatening, chronic, and terminal conditions. An example of its application in a non-lifethreatening situation is the choice one makes about dental procedures. For some, tooth extraction is preferable to root canal, for others the opposite is true—and the choice is not confined to clinical criteria.

Certainly the clearest example of the use of the distinction in terminal conditions is the decision about forgoing life support: deciding about "Do Not Resuscitate" orders and removing life support. These are the most difficult cases, where patients, families, and caregivers grapple with poor prognoses, and so on.

In the final analysis, this distinction is precisely what radically separates these sorts of decisions from the siren song of euthanasia: a decision to forgo extraordinary means rests on a recognition that the means of preserving life or restoring health are no longer beneficial, are no longer useful, or are too burdensome. It is not a decision that the life of the patient is no longer one worthy of being lived.

Rev. Russell E. Smith, S.T.D.
Theological and Health Care Consultant
Diocese of Richmond, Virginia

The Catholic Health Care Institution

Service to the Community

Not-for-Profit Catholic Health Care

Along with its pursuit of what might be considered its "sectarian" interest of proclaiming the gospel of the Lord Jesus, the Catholic health ministry is rooted in a commitment to promote and defend human dignity. Its focus is outward, toward the person and the community. This concentration on the person is more than a public relations ploy or even a preference. It is mandated by the Church's ethical directives:

> A Catholic institutional health care service is a community that provides health care to those in need of it.... In accord with its mission, Catholic health care should distinguish itself by service to and advocacy for those people whose social condition puts them at the margins of our society and makes them particularly vulnerable to discrimination: the poor; the uninsured and the underinsured; children and the unborn; single parents; the elderly; those with incurable diseases and chemical dependencies; racial minorities; immigrants and refugees (*Ethical and Religious Directives for Catholic Health Care Services* [1995], nn. 1, 3).

The Catholic health ministry teaches that health care is a social good rendered in response to basic human need. Like education, adequate access to health care is essential for individuals to achieve their full human potential. Health care services are often provided when we are sick, preoccupied with worry, and highly dependent on a trustful relationship with professionals. Given its special status, health care's primary end or essential purpose should be a cured patient, a comforted person, and a healthier community, *not earning a profit* or return on capital for shareholders. I am convinced that the same should be said for all health care delivery in our nation.

What corporate structure can best focus on the needs of the people served by a hospital and, most importantly, on the needs of those who are most vulnerable: a not-for-profit hospital or a publicly traded investor-owned corporation? I submit that both logic and accumulated evidence point to the former.

By definition, investor-owned institutions have as their primary fiduciary duty to ensure a reasonable return for shareholders. Most of these shareholders do not live in the community where a hospital is located, and when the expectation of an ever-growing return on investment is not met, the capital is withdrawn and reinvested in other enterprises. Moving resources to other more lucrative investments may not be wrong when the commodity in question is a computer, camera, or car. Those managing pension funds and the investments of wealthy individuals have a duty to maximize their return. I am not condemning this practice. It is the nature of publicly-traded, investor-owned institutions. As I have said, however, health care is different, and communities are wise to treat it that way.

Health care is too important to risk on the long-term incentives that accompany investor-owned health care. In order to conclude that an investor-owned hospital that serves a local community benefits the community, you must believe that it will defy the expectations that we have of investor-owned institutions in every other area of the economy.

Ordered to the Community

The distinguishing feature of not-for-profit institutions is that legally and morally they owe their duty to the community they serve. Unlike investor-owned organizations, they are not designed for the purpose of providing a return on capital to shareholders. For that reason, they have a loyalty to the community that is not called into question when return on capital falls below a certain preordained percentage.

This analysis is not merely theory based on the fiduciary duties of investor-owned and not-for-profit hospitals. It has been borne out in numerous studies of investor-owned institutions throughout the country. Admittedly, there are studies on both sides of this issue. Investor-owned health care institutions question the methodology and the conclusions of the studies cited herein. Likewise, the not-for-profit community questions the conclusions of studies cited by investor-owned institutions. I believe, however, that it is important to know that reputable academics have found that investor-owned institutions tend to reduce access to "unprofitable" care and raise prices for their services.

According to the Georgia state health planning agency, in 1995 not-for-profit hospitals in Georgia provided nearly three times more uncompensated care on a per-bed basis than investor-owned hospitals (Weissenstien, *Modern Healthcare* [May 5, 1997], 20). Four well-respected scholars recently examined twenty studies of comparative community benefit and came to the following conclusion: "Nonprofit hospitals provide significantly more community benefits than for-profit hospitals provide. The differences are more evident when comparisons are made across hospitals within states ..." (Claxton, Feder, Shactman, and Altman, *Health Affairs* [March/April 1997], 18). Other studies have shown that not-for-profit hospitals provide substantially higher levels of charity care than for-profits.

This inevitable erosion of community benefits in an investor-owned health care organization is not hard to understand. Investor-owned institutions respond to the demand of shareholders. If it is a choice between the bottom line and a patient who cannot pay, management has a legal obligation to shareholders from outside the community to favor the former. Not-for-profit hospitals, on the other hand, owe their fiduciary duty to the person seeking care, not to a shareholder thousands of miles away.

The Problem of For-Profit Health Care

In studying the contribution of not-for-profit hospitals to the common good, we cannot allow business executives to confuse the narrow concept of "charity care" with the broader notion of "community benefit." Not-for-profit providers offer more benefit to their communities than simply providing "charity care." They have the mission and the freedom to provide more unprofitable "essential community services," like assistance for those with HIV, burn care, facilities for low birth weight neonates, high-risk obstetrics, and trauma care. They also offer more positive services accentuating the creation of "healthier communities."

In addition to issues associated with charity care, studies show that investor-owned hospitals tend to raise charges and increase prices faster and higher than not-for-profits. This can be done in a variety of ways, some of which might be alarming to those committed to looking after the patient first. One of those methods will be raising prices to the surrounding community. Another strategy is to reduce "unprofitable" services. The third and most likely scenario is that an investor-owned institution will be forced to do both.

For example, in Virginia for-profit hospitals had 17.1% higher costs per admission in 1993 than not-for-profits, even after data were adjusted for the taxes paid by for-profits (Lisa Scott, *Modern Healthcare* [May 5, 1997], 20), who reports on a study by Shukla, Pestian, and Clement of Virginia Commonwealth University). According to one recent study of acute care hospitals, for-profit institutions had higher adjusted costs per discharge than did private not-for-profit or public hospitals. In Georgia, adjusted for case mix, charges averaged from 14 to 57% higher in investor-owned hospitals (Julie Trocchio, *Nursing Policy Forum* 17 [July/August 1997], who cites *Georgia Not-For-Profit Hospital: Analysis of Hospital Community Benefits*, prepared for Georgia Alliance for the Not-For-Profit Hospital, by Parker, Hudson, Rainer, and Dobbs [1994]).

In Texas, Medicare pays nearly 10% more for care originating at investor-owned Columbia hospitals than at other hospitals (*New York Times* [March 28, 1997], C15). According to another recent article, Tenet HealthSystem's own St. Joseph Hospital in Omaha—formerly, a not-for-profit Catholic hospital—"has hiked its prices five times in two years, yielding large profits and making it perhaps the highest priced hospital in town. Yet, it will not admit uninsured patients for nonemergency testing and surgery, forcing doctors to refer them to other facilities" (Harris Meyer, *Hospitals and Health Networks* [July 20, 1997], 38).

What Motivation for Health Care Providers?

While there is, and will continue to be, a rigorous debate in the professional literature about the true impact of investor-owned institutions on their communities, I believe that this uncertainty should lead us to step back and ask the more fundamental question: *What economic incentives would you want to drive the health care you receive*? The late Cardinal Joseph Bernardin answered this question powerfully:

> To be sure, we expect our physician to earn a good living and our hospital to be economically viable, but when it comes to *our* case, we do not expect them to be motivated mainly by self-interest. When it comes to *our* coronary bypass or our hip replacement or *our* child's cancer treatment, we expect them to be professional in the original sense of that term—motivated primarily by patient need, not economic self-interest. We have no comparable expectation—nor should we—of General Motors or Wal-Mart. ("Making the Case for Not-for-Profit Healthcare," speech to Harvard Business School Club of Chicago [January 12, 1995], 2).

This is an issue we must continue to analyze. Catholic health care, also, must become more effective in finding objective criteria for communicating its community benefit. In a nondefensive manner we have to continue to ask the question: "In the long run, will an investor-focused hospital continue to put patients and the community first?"

Rev. Michael D. Place, S.T.D.
President and Chief Executive Officer
Catholic Health Association
St. Louis, Missouri

Technological Achievement or Patient Health?

In the past two decades, medical technology has undergone an unparalleled growth. Procedures done today were the stuff of science fiction only a short time ago. Nearly every month, a news story headlines another "medical breakthrough." One of the disconcerting byproducts of this rapid proliferation of scientific technology has been the often late and almost always anticli mactic cry of some medical ethicists. It goes something like "maybe we should think this technology's effects through before trying it or continuing with it." In these moments, an apparent conflict is sensed between medicine and ethics. The conflict is produced because, to many modern minds, good medicine is simply equated with good science. The result may be an accusatory retort that medical ethics is getting in the way of progress and, thereby, ultimately hurting the patients we serve. The real conflict here is not between science and ethics, but between competing value systems: one which prizes technological achievement as an appropriate end of medical endeavor and another which emphasizes something perhaps far less tangible, objective, or exciting—the health of the individual.

Medicine as a Cognitive Art

Medicine is neither science, nor ethics, nor scientism. Scientism is decidedly not science but a value system which sees all things in the limited framework of scientific progress. Some believe that what can be done, should be done; or, at the very least, will be done—so why wring our hands and fret about it? In contrast, doctors, nurses, and other health care providers must always note the difference between doing something and doing something right. Moments of apparent conflict like these, when medicine seems jostled by what can be done and what *should* be done, are the true testing grounds for the ethical practice of medicine. When we question whether or not sound ethics can hurt our patients, we simultaneously ask, "Why do we do what we do as health care providers?"

The answer is found in the *telos* of medicine, i.e., the end towards which medicine is ordered. If medicine were a science, then, like all sciences, its *telos* would be knowledge, i.e., an organized system of truths which would reveal a specific part of the universe to us. For example, chemistry seeks to explain and understand the nature of the elements and their interactions, biology is concerned with knowing all that can be known about life and living organisms, etc. Clearly, all of us who care for patients understand that this is not really what medicine is about.

Although we use knowledge gained from the sciences, we are most concerned with its application to an individual person to achieve a desired end. If medicine were simply a technology, then technological achievement would be its obvious goal. The ability to apply new and varied techniques in an ever more efficient manner would rule the medical decision. But the end, or purpose, of medicine is neither science (knowledge) nor technology (process); rather it is *health*, and most specifically the health of individual human persons. As difficult as it may be to categorize what health is, we know that it exists as a *good* of living bodies.

As health care providers, we utilize knowledge and technology to help our patients attain and maintain health or become healthier. This specific end point of health is unique for each patient, so we must individualize the knowledge and technology we use in arriving at the advice we give patients. Health care providers are, in essence, making choices about what is good for particular persons. Making choices about what is good for particular persons is moral work.

Thus, medicine is the moral application of knowledge, often via technology, for the health of an individual human person. Far from being a science or technology, medicine could best be classified as a cognitive art (see Pellegrino and Thomasma, *What is Medicine? A Philosophical Basis of Medical Practice* [New York: Oxford University Press, 1981], esp. chap. 8, 170–191).

Since medicine does not share similar ends with the disciplines it relies on to produce its results, there should be no true conflict between them and medicine. Conflicts arise when we lose sight of the goal of medicine and try to force other purposes onto it, obscuring its true end.

Reliance of Medicine on Many Disciplines

Claiming that good science can make for bad medicine or that good ethics can have the same negative result misses the point. Medicine relies on various sciences, ethics, and a host of other disciplines to reach its end. It is most served by using the best each discipline has to offer. As an analogy, it is unlikely that using the best paint and brushes accounts in large measure for the quality of a work of art. Poor paint and poor brushes are generally detrimental to producing a masterpiece of lasting value. Similarly, in medicine, using poor science and/or poor ethics will likely result in poor medicine, because part of the skill of this cognitive art is knowing the necessary material for making decisions.

The other part of the skill is completely different. To carry our artist analogy further, it involves knowing the canvas, knowing what it will allow or reject, in other words, knowing what its capacity is. As health care providers, we are to know what our patients are capable of as examples of the human species and as unique human persons. This knowledge must go beyond the biological, because we know human persons to be much more than that.

The next to the last expression of a medical decision is the suggestion of a recommended course of action for a particular patient to undertake. (N.B. Even when it is the health care providers who take the action, they do so with the explicit or implicit consent of the patient.) Ultimately, this recommendation is further worked upon through processes of consultation and informed consent to produce the best course of action that the particular patient finds acceptable. There can be little doubt that a health care provider's intimate knowledge of his patients is vital to expanding or limiting the range of options.

One of the most important functions of medical ethics is aiding the health care provider in assessing the capacities of the patient. Catholic medical ethics, with its firm grounding in the teleology of the human person and in natural law, is particularly useful in helping us understand why some technologies are out of touch with the inherent dignity of the human person as a creature who reflects the likeness of the Creator. Furthermore, the emphasis on individual circumstance, which is so important to the Catholic understanding of free choice and moral obligation, goes beyond any impersonal "victory" that modern technology may force upon the person.

Even if health care providers use more than science in medical decision making, that alone will not insure good medicine. As noted above, poor ingredients will produce poor results. The ethics, and all the other disciplines we use to formulate our advice, must be sound. When a colleague or patient senses conflict, we need to address this perception. Our proposed advice to a patient (i.e., the medical decision prior to instruction of the patient) may indeed be wrong for any number of reasons.

Questions to Be Asked

A series of questions should immediately come to mind when we are faced with the assertion that our ethics is hurting someone:

1. Are the facts of the case established and verified, or are they in dispute? Are our questioners aware of these facts?
2. Is our science faulty? Is our ethics faulty? Have we consulted with others for their views? Can we support our advice (medical decision) logically and with evidence?
3. Does our advice violate any principle of our profession?
4. Does our advice violate any principle of our own informed conscience?
5. Have we communicated our advice clearly and understandably?

Careful answers to these questions should allow us to find and correct errors in knowledge, process, and expression of our medical decisions while complementing the value system most apropos to medical decision making, i.e., one based in the teleology of the human person and in the *telos* of medicine.

Charles E. Cavagnaro III, M.D.
Belchertown Medical Center
Belchertown, Massachusetts

Establishing a Hospital Ethics Committee

Ethics committees are among the most effective forums for promoting human dignity and the common good in the health care setting, and for exploring the practical implications of various methodologies, cases, and principles for health care organization and practice. Directive thirty-seven of the *Ethical and Religious Directives for Catholic Health Care Services* (1995) states that

> An ethics committee or some alternate form of ethical consultation should be available to assist by advising on particular ethical situations, by offering educational opportunities, and by reviewing and recommending policies. To these ends, there should be appropriate standards for medical ethical consultation within a particular diocese that will respect the diocesan bishop's pastoral responsibilities as well as assist members of ethics committees to be familiar with Catholic medical ethics and, in particular, these *Directives*.

Directive thirty-seven can pertain to institutional ethics committees, system committees, a consultation service, a multisystem committee, a diocesan committee, or any combination of these.

The directive encourages appropriate standards for medical-ethical consultation that respect the local bishop's pastoral role. Catholic-sponsored health care is an apostolate of the Church, and as such, lies within the bishop's pastoral jurisdiction. The bishop's pastoral role can be summarized as the principal governor, preacher, teacher, and priest of the local Church. (The Greek word for bishop, *episkopos*, literally means "overseer.")

The Need for Committees

The Church's teaching does not demand that a Catholic health care organization have an ethics committee. Neither do the *Directives*. Directive thirty-seven simply states that "an ethics committee *or some alternate form of ethical consultation should be available*" (emphasis added). However, every Catholic-sponsored health care service *does* have a moral obligation to promote the Church's teaching and to commit itself to human dignity and the common good. That vision, summarized but not exhausted in the *Directives*, has far reaching implications for the physician-patient relationship, for spiritual care, employee relations, marketing practices, beginning-of-life and end-of-life care, health care partnerships, and other matters.

The appropriateness of ethics committees as one means of imparting the Catholic vision of health care is implied elsewhere in the *Directives*. Directive five requires that "appropriate instruction regarding the *Directives*" be given to all employees and to those with staff privileges. Directive nine states that "employees of a Catholic health care institution must respect and uphold the religious mission of the institution" and "maintain professional standards and promote the institution's commitment to human dignity and the common good." Directive twenty-eight states that a patient or surrogate "should have access to medical and moral information and counseling" for conscience formation, and that "the free and informed health care decision of the person or the person's surrogate is to be followed so long as it does not contradict Catholic principles." The ethics committee is an ideal forum for gathering people from all sectors of the institution to address these objectives.

Roles of the Committee

Directive thirty-seven identifies three roles for the ethics committee: advisory or consultative, educational, and policy review and development. The educational is arguably the most important. Committee members are responsible first and foremost for educating themselves. New ethics committees perhaps should refrain from providing consultation service for a year or more until the consulting members possess: an appropriate understanding of the purpose and role of the ethics committee and of the ethics consultation service; a broad understanding of ethical and legal principles; a working knowledge of classic cases, case studies, and case methods; and a thorough understanding of the ethical policies of the institution, including the *Directives*. New members to an existing committee might participate in consultations as observers only until they possess such qualifications.

Many may think of the ethics consultative service as the primary function of an ethics committee, but it is rarely the most consuming work. Committee members often share their insights informally with their coworkers—counseling them, in effect, on important ethical issues in the health care environment. When the consultation service is formally accessed, the committee should use the opportunity to foster appropriate decision-making processes, clarify responsibilities, and promote a heightened awareness and understanding of human dignity, the *Directives*, and institutional policies. The consultation service is principally an educational function that facilitates appropriate moral decisions and decision making among patients, surrogates, physicians, nurses, and other caregivers.

Like the consultative function of an ethics committee, its policy review and development role is also educational in character. The administration should make liberal use of the ethics committee for help in reviewing and in developing policies on clinical care, employee relations, and even managed care contracts. The work of the ethics committee should relate to the day-to-day lives and ministry of its members. The committee will founder if the members see little or no apparent relationship between the committee's work and their patients.

Representation and Membership

The committee should have a well-balanced representation from medical and nursing staffs as well as from pastoral/spriritual care, social work, discharge planning, and other areas directly involved in patient care. A health law attorney can be an effective addition so long as he or she does not place risk concerns above ethical concerns. Not all members need to be moral theologians, but someone well acquainted with the moral methodology and teaching of the Catholic Church is vital to the committee's mission. An administrative liaison also should serve. The progress and success of a committee depend upon its composition and reporting structure. In a Catholic-sponsored organization, the committee should be appointed by and report directly to the administration. A committee that does not have the full support of the administration is doomed to failure or mediocrity at best.

Committee members should possess certain qualifications: an interest in ethics and a willingness to contribute to committee responsibilities and to attend meetings; an appropriate educational or professional background; practical employment or volunteer pursuits that will contribute to the work of the committee; an appreciation of and willingness to support the Catholic health ministry, in accord with the *Directives*; a willingness to articulate the Catholic moral tradition; an openness to the ethical wisdom found in other religious traditions and secular culture; sound moral character and the ability to respect others' opinions; a commitment to confidentiality; and a willingness to disclose any existing or potential conflicts of interest.

Most committee members will not be ethical "experts." Nor is this necessarily desirable. Above all, members must be committed to the mission of the institution, respectful and open, willing and able to learn, and ready to share what they have learned with others.

Nor is it necessary or even desirable for all members of the committee to be Catholic, though it is arguably prudent for practicing Catholics to hold some of the key positions on the committee, when possible. Other religious perspectives, however, can greatly enrich the ethical discourse and contribute to a committee's effectiveness in responding to questions raised by employees, professional staffs, and patients who come from diverse religious backgrounds.

Who Assumes Responsibility?

Twenty-four years after Karen Quinlan, most reflection on the proper functions of ethics committees has maintained that decision-making authority rests within the physician-patient relationship. The *Directives* offer a balanced model of the professional-patient relationship as a partnership of moral equals, albeit unequal in expertise.

> The health care professional has the knowledge and experience to pursue the goals of healing, the maintenance of health, and the compassionate care of the dying, taking into account the patient's convictions and spiritual needs, and the moral responsibilities of all concerned. The person in need of health care depends on the skill of the health care provider to assist in preserving life and promoting health of body, mind, and spirit. The patient, in turn, has a responsibility to use these physical and mental resources in the service of moral and spiritual goals to the best of his or her ability. (*Directives*, Part Three, Introduction.)

A consultation service must not exercise the moral authority that rightly belongs to the physician and to the patient, or to those professionals and others immediately involved in the patient's care. If decision-making powers were exercised by ethics committees, they in effect could distance or remove moral responsibility from those most accountable for the patient's welfare. This could have the additional effect of undermining the committee's credibility among medical staffs.

Should committee members "parrot" Church teaching or should they speak their own minds? The Church holds that, in principle, the teachings of faith and reason do not contradict each other. All truth has but one source—God the Creator of all. Moreover, there are certain kinds of truth for which the Church cannot claim any special competency. For example, the Church claims no unique insights into the biology of the human body or medical science. However, drawing from the teachings and example of Jesus, from the experience of the lived faith, and from the natural wisdom gained from various disciplines, the Church does claim unique insight into the dignity of the human person. These teachings have moral implications for the use of science and the practice of medicine—particularly when these fall under the sponsorship of the Church. In light of the above, anyone serving on the ethics committee should speak his or her mind freely and respectfully for the sake of seeking deeper understanding and possible common ground. When there is agreement on the need to promote human dignity and the common good, then the rich diversity of professional and community experience and expertise that each member brings to the committee will add insight to every other member and enrich the ministry of the organization as a whole.

Daniel O'Brien, Ph.D.
Vice-President, Ethics
Ascension Health
St. Louis, Missouri

Respect for the Patient

Confidentiality and Truth-Telling

The principle of confidentiality is the bedrock of the therapeutic relationship. The confidence one places in a healing relationship goes beyond the importance of keeping secrets to encompass a whole series of trusts, without which the health care professional loses both the authority and the power to heal. The degree to which these trusts are freely given and conscientiously responded to largely determines the success of the relationship.

The confidences patients place in their caregivers are of four major categories, best described in terms of rights.

1. Patients have a right to confidentiality, that is, that those to whom they have legitimately entrusted their secrets, treat such with respect.
2. Patients have a right to privacy, that is, that no secret will be unwillingly, unnecessarily, or unwittingly extracted from them.
3. Patients have a right to hear the truth, as it is known and as it pertains to their particular situation.
4. Patients have a right that information given about them be as accurate as possible.

To each of these rights there is a corresponding obligation which the Christian virtues of justice and charity demand from the caregivers. Professionals violating or failing these confidences injure their patients and seriously damage the credibility of their profession, negatively affecting the common good.

The Limits of Confidentiality

Health care professionals hear the private lives and innermost thoughts of their patients. From earliest times, the obligation to keep knowledge about patients that was "not fitting" to be spoken an inviolable secret weighed heavily on professional consciences (see the "Hippocratic Oath," trans. L. Edelstein, *Ancient Medicine* [Baltimore: The Johns Hopkins University Press, 1967], 6).

The keeping of secrets, well-founded in both religious and secular philosophies, has always been regarded as sacrosanct in medicine, often compared to the seal of confession, albeit erroneously, to underscore its gravity.

In modern society, we now recognize a number of instances where other equally grave matters may outweigh the obligation to keep a patient's secret. Some are imposed by the state, such as knowledge about child or elder abuse or in certain cases of communicable diseases. Others are imposed by morality, such as knowledge that would preserve the common good, save a life, or rescue another's or one's own reputation or freedom. Items may be publicly known or not validly owned by the person presenting them as secrets. These are not legitimate secrets, and there is no obligation to keep them in confidence. Entrusted secrets also lose their claim on the professional when they are publicly revealed or become common knowledge. Some moralists (e.g., Orville Griese, *Catholic Identity in Health Care: Principles and Practice* [Braintree, MA: The Pope John Center, 1987], 355) propose that one can reveal an entrusted secret if one can be justifiably certain that the individual involved would give consent to do so if he knew of the situation. While this may be morally correct in theory, in practice we can almost never be justifiably certain of consent.

The obligation to keep secrets extends to all forms of communication, including the written and electronic record. It also extends to all those who extend the work of the health care professional such as transcriptionists, billing agents, lab technicians, and a host of others. The breaching of confidentiality accounts for a sizable number of professional malpractice cases. While some are test cases involving the borders of the issue, in which one principle conflicts with another (common good vs. confidentiality), most breaches remain everyday lapses, usually unintentional, and the result of carelessness. In an age of computerized medicine, particular burdens are placed on confidentiality. Computer hackers can enter the most secure computer databases. Medical computerized information is used by so many persons that serious breaches are bound to occur. One can reasonably wonder if anything can be assured of confidentiality once placed "on-line." We may need to think about what information should be kept back in some other form, apart from the computerized chart.

Free Consent

For these reasons, the right to privacy is confined to a patient's right to protect knowledge about one's self and family (cf. *Communio et progressio* [*Pastoral Instruction on the Means of Social Communication*], n. 42, in *Vatican Council II: The Conciliar and Post Conciliar Documents*, ed. Austin Flannery, O.P. [Northport, New York: Costello Publishing Co., 1992], 307). Giving up private information even to a health care professional should be done freely and with an understanding of how that information will be used. Patients should never be forced to reveal things about themselves, even if maintaining secrecy causes therapeutic difficulties. For example, a patient is not obligated to reveal his sexual orientation, even if it may help to make the diagnosis and aid treatment. Similarly, patients who withhold private information must realize the danger they face by doing so and accept this. Before a procedure is undertaken (e.g., hypnosis), mental health professionals must inform patients what information may be revealed by it. The information revealed may be startling even to the patient, and must be treated with utmost caution. The current controversy over repressed memories and their validity as accurate representations of previous events bears witness to the sensitive nature of one's innermost thoughts, dreams, and memories. Patients participating in research retain their right to privacy throughout the activity. Every privately held thought, secret, or memory revealed requires a new consent, as each must be revealed freely, knowingly, and willingly.

Patients in Vulnerable Situations

The basic moral tenet to speak truthfully and not lie binds professionals even within the context of their special duties. While lying is never permissible, telling the whole, cold, and sometimes hard truth to persons in vulnerable situations is a subject of controversy. Many professionals argue that revealing grave diagnoses or prognoses can cause patients added anguish and hopelessness, ultimately hastening their demise or leading to despair. Thus, these professionals say, the burdens outweigh the benefits. In most of these situations, patients already know or suspect something is seriously wrong. By withholding the truth in grave situations we breach the trust placed in us by our promise to help. Honesty and candor in these situations are almost always helpful, and evidence increasingly supports this. It allows patients to prepare for the hardships ahead, and can be the impetus for a healing peace for patients and families as they refocus their priorities and shift energies away from maintaining facades to more important endeavors.

The obligation to tell the truth is not a license for harshness or insensitivity. Caring, empathy, and gentleness are always possible even with the worst of news. Health care professionals should always be about the work of healing; even in helpless situations hope remains despite its change in focus. Reserving part of the truth remains an acceptable moral alternative, if one judges that the whole truth, even if revealed in the best possible way, would be too burdensome and result in harm. An example would be telling a patient he has an untreatable malignancy, but reserving the details of its extent for a more suitable time. There is no obligation to tell the whole truth all in one instance. The timing of revelations remains part of the art of healing, and should never be deceptive or consciously misleading.

Language and Accuracy

The language we use with patients and the advice we give them are other areas where truth-telling pertains. In medicine, it is possible to tell the whole truth in such a way that the patient hasn't a clue about what it means. This kind of *medspeak* is useless and annoying to patients; furthermore, it shirks the responsibility we have to inform patients. Asking patients if they understand what we have told them is as important to fulfilling our obligation to truth-telling as it is to informed consent. These two principles rest on good communication skills. In advising patients, we need to be truthful and unambiguous in our instructions. In some cases, formal notification in writing may be needed to reach this goal. For example, it is not sufficient to say that continued smoking may lead to poor health; we must tell the truth about all it can do, including leading to premature death.

Accuracy is usually not thought of as part of the principle of confidentiality. However, it is a corollary to truth-telling. Confidentiality avoids inappropriately telling others the truth about the patient. As such, accuracy pertains mostly to the keeping of medical records and the correspondence that revolves around them. The medical chart is a compendium of information about the patient's health care and includes subjective and objective data, observations, correspondence, etc. Negative statements in the record about the patient should be rare and based on objective data. For example, recording that someone is "noncompliant" should be followed by evidence. Informing the patient that such an entry is being made gives him an opportunity to respond and may shed light on the reasons for the negative behavior, thereby creating an occasion for change. The medical record is often a source for information having insurance, compensation, or legal significance. Good record keeping can make a difference, and in justice the complete findings of any professional encounter need to be available to support or refute claims arising about the patient, his condition, and his care.

The Christian health care professional may find the obligations imposed by confidentiality burdensome at times, but they pale in comparison to the joy we have in knowing we are giving witness to the great dignity of the human person. In keeping faith with those entrusted to our care, we mirror the covenant God has made with his people. In keeping their secrets while we try to aid them, we reflect the work of Christ (" A bruised reed he will not break, a smoldering wick he will not quench" [Matt.12:20]). We strive to create a relationship between patient and professional that becomes, as in the vision of the Holy Father, John Paul II, "a real meeting between two free people ... between a trust and a conscience" ("The Person, Not Science, Is the Measure," Address to 81st Congress of the Italian Society of Internal Medicine and 82nd Congress of the Italian Society of General Surgery (October 27, 1980), in *Sacred in All Its Forms* [Boston: St. Paul Editions, 1984], 325).

Charles E. Cavagnaro III, M.D.
Belchertown Medical Center
Belchertown, Massachusetts

Justice as a Social Virtue

According to the long tradition of Catholic ethics, justice is a cardinal virtue. More specifically, it is the moral virtue that consists in the constant and firm will to give God and neighbor their due (*Catechism of the Catholic Church*, n. 1807). Verbally, of course, virtue suggests several things: strength, moral excellence, the perfection of an inclination or power of the soul. What inclination or power then does justice strengthen and bring to perfection? At what excellence does it aim? What are its roots?

Justice and History

Justice has been thought to be many things, but the Catholic conception originates in Sacred Scripture (revelation) and in the work of the pre-Christian philosophers reflecting on natural law (reason). Again and again, the Old Testament uses the expression "the just man" to refer to the one who is complete in goodness before God and man. The New Testament teaches the completeness of justice in such passages as Luke's reference (17:7–10) to the "unprofitable" servant who is to profess that he has only done his duty (what he owes his master).

The first focused philosophical treatment of justice as a virtue dates back to the work of Plato, whose *Republic* is dedicated to this theme, and who sees justice as due social order. Previously, justice was known almost intuitively by the quasi-legendary "seven sages" of Greece, who knew that it was contemporaneous with mankind and that it was evenhanded (Thales), that it was universally and mutually owed among persons (Solon), and that it was rule by the just, and exclusion of the wicked, that makes a state good (Pittacus). These ancient sayings are found to be worthy of record for posterity by Plutarch, Diogenes Laertius, and Strobaeus. Subsequent to Plato, Aristotle, his greatest disciple and "the mind of the school," taught that justice required those acts which benefit the natural political society, and that it respects the proportionate equality between excess and defect in acts of giving to others.

In the *Summa Theologiae*, St. Thomas Aquinas finds the native compatibility of the revealed and reasoned accounts of justice, teaching with Aristotle that justice in action is rendering that which is owed to each person. In the *Summa contra Gentiles* (II, 28–9), he adds that God's creation of persons is the genesis of justice because creation is the genesis of subjects to whom justice is owed, but that creation is a pure act of free giving, rather than a preexisting obligation of God to man.

With the radical intellectual and practical revolution of the sixteenth and seventeenth centuries, the conscious, deliberate rejection of Aristotle and Catholic Christianity motivated a new doctrine of justice—in short, one that is artificial and in this sense arbitrary. The most salient features of the new conception of justice are that it 1) is manmade; 2) proceeds from willing rather than discovery; 3) is at root subjective; 4) removes men from the (unenviable) conflictual condition of nature; and 5) serves the ends of the politically powerful. This description of justice generates the modern notions of the equation of knowledge with power, the immanence of human destiny, and the combative character of reality, human and otherwise (see, e.g., Bacon, Hobbes, Locke, Rousseau, Darwin, and Bertrand Russell).

As Giuseppe Mazzini observed in the nineteenth century, ideas rule the world, and these are the ideas which have won the day and are incarnate in the modern world. We do well to remember that out of Hegel's absolute state emerged a driving and forceful idea which fueled the Third Reich, that this was further fed by a radical subjectivism of morals (as in Mussolini's regime), and that the Marxism which until only recently governed a third of the world's population was the same Marxism which led Stalin to murder millions of his Ukrainian peasants, Mao to kill in excess of fifty million of his countrymen, and Pol Pot to carry out a similar slaughter in Cambodia's killing fields. Given the healthy insight of common sense that modern "Justice" is anything but this disastrous outcome, what indeed is justice? What, in other words, is the alternative to the theories which were generated by modern thinkers in their revolt against the Bible, the Church, and the classical philosophies of Plato and Aristotle?

The Virtue of Justice

St. Thomas defines justice as the virtue which is a constant and firm will to render what is due to each man (ST II-II, 58.1). Among his references in this article are Aristotle, St. Augustine, and St. Anselm, and, even while the setting for the article is entirely theological, his treatment is primarily natural, from reason. In saying that justice is a firm and constant determination of the will, there is a reaffirmation of the doctrine that the genus of virtue is a habit, i.e., a constant way of acting developed by repetition, practice and cultivation. (How, after all, does one become a good dancer, but by dancing?) But the repetition is not by rote, and in fact cannot be by rote, for no two sets of conditions requiring just action are identical. What a virtue does is to enhance and strengthen a natural human proclivity, in this case the inclination to society. What the virtue of justice develops in this way is the will in its relation to God and man—the universal ability, corresponding to reason, to desire and direct one's course of action and life by choosing what is good in relation to others.

Consider, as an illustration, the selfish will of a young child. He knows and desires and pursues good, but in a restricted way, i.e., the good for himself. With good guidance he can also come to recognize the legitimate claims of others to what is good, and this can "open" from the singular instance of self to the entire social realm.

Thus, as the will is the principle of rational direction towards the good in life, so the virtue of justice emerges to be reasonable (grounded in natural law and reason, and thus a matter of knowledge rather than feeling) and to be an excellence and perfection in one's relations with others. In short, the relationship between justice and natural law, man and society, is reciprocal, each contributing to the betterment of the other.

Three Kinds of Justice

The manifestations of justice are of three basic kinds: commutative, legal, and distributive. Each is a kind of moral and social order of persons in a social whole. Each is a form of indebtedness; and each requires that it be "supported and realized" in and by the just man.

Nevertheless, they differ. Commutative justice characterizes the social order of individual to individual; distributive justice governs the order of obligations proceeding from the social whole (e.g., the state) to its membership; and "legal" or "general" justice obliges the individuals in a social whole to serve the building up of the common good of that whole. Commutative justice is determinable by a disinterested third party, who could be, for example, anyone reading a contract; commutative justice is largely a matter of simple numerical equality, as St. Thomas calls it, following the usage of Aristotle—say, a book for a certain number of dollars. The other two forms of justice require a specially-positioned person, namely, one who knows and serves the whole.

The equality of justice here is "proportional," again following the usage of St. Thomas after Aristotle. It is determined not merely according to material and established demands, but also according to the exigencies of the common good, which is both material and nonmaterial. Thus, in making recompense for damages, not only financial loss but also suffering incurred, ability to pay, and the other needs of society drawing upon its stock of common good must enter into consideration.

In the modern conception, rights are fabricated by those in power, vary according to the will of society, and are primarily characteristics by which individuals are enabled to make demands on one another. This yields a society of self-centered expectations. By contrast, St. Thomas sees the existence of rights as indeed prior to the obligations of justice, both of which are natural, knowable, and unchanging. Rights precede justice as a bull's-eye in a target precedes an accurate shot. God created man as one to whom acts of justice are owed. Before his creation, however, man was not rightfully owed the privilege of being created. Thus, creation is that act whereby something becomes due to man from man. In the order of reality, rights are prior to justice. In the order of knowledge, the obligations of justice are known to be owed mutually, and the "right" which demands them is known by inference. Moreover, the rights and obligations of justice imply one another—for John to owe Peter $100 is to say that Peter has the right to his $100 from John.

Justice in Just Persons

Finally, one must stress that there is no justice apart from just persons, and that for a person to be just, he must integrate in himself all the cardinal virtues; not only justice but also fortitude, temperance, and especially prudence. Indeed, so important is justice that in the carrying out of any act of virtue there is the fulfillment of a debt that is owed to God, self, or others, and so all good action is suffused by justice, and there can be no moral good apart from justice.

Theodore P. Rebard, Ph.D.
Assistant Professor of Philosophy
University of St. Thomas
Houston, Texas

Human Experimentation and Research

How do physicians find out what is a safe and effective treatment for sick human beings? One way is to consider the accumulated medical practice of the past. Usually by trial and error the physicians of the past determined what was effective for curing one or another disease condition of their patients. Of course, errors were made, but lessons were learned and passed on to the medical community. Some of this past research was to a degree systematic, some was haphazard; much depended on the physician's previous training and experience. Generally, such attempts were motivated by the desire of the physicians to be of help to their patients. Gradually, the armamentarium of the practicing physician was increased by the accumulation of experiences of physicians throughout the world which was shared by word of mouth and in medical literature.

Past Experience

In the past new medications and procedures were the result of serendipity and/or careful observation. Thus, for example, one version has it that quinine was discovered by the observation that Peruvian Indians would drink water accumulated at the base of the cinchona tree. William Withering (1685) noted that a brew made up of some 100 plants was successful in treating dropsy. He discovered the plant responsible was *Digitalis purpurea*. The immunosuppressive drug cyclosporine was discovered as a product of a fungus found in Norwegian arctic soil. In our day it is now a common practice of pharmaceutical companies to investigate native medicinal plants for their active medicinal components in order to identify them chemically, which then often permits synthesis of the active principle(s) as well as more effective clinical studies.

Gradually, a more systematic approach was introduced into the means of bringing new knowledge into medical practice: *controlled* human experimentation. Among the first to use treated control groups in the testing of new treatments was the English naval surgeon James Lind, who in 1747 took twelve scurvy patients aboard his ship, divided them into six groups of two, and placed each pair on a different dietary regimen. The group that received oranges and lemons showed the most improvement (see Curtis L. Meinert with Susan Tomascia, *Clinical Trials* [New York: Oxford University Press, 1986], 5).

Because the primary focus of the early research on human subjects was on the *scientific* aspect of the research, not much attention was paid to the *ethical* aspects, particularly the rights of the human subjects of that research. Not that these were ignored—some researchers had a very strong sense of what was ethically correct or wrong in human research. But there was very little official attention paid to the subject, probably under the presumption that the individual medical researcher was ethically upright and could be depended upon to do the ethically right thing. Also, for many in the medical field, particularly outside of the Catholic community, ethics was often interpreted primarily to mean etiquette, a set of rules, written and unwritten, which while it dictated the relationship that ought to prevail between and among physicians, also proclaimed the priority of a patient's well-being among other concerns of the physician.

The Nuremberg Code

However, confidence in a code of honor, that is, in this kind of gentlemen's agreement among physicians that their knowledge and professional actions would be used only for the good of their patients, was shattered when the revelations of medical atrocities which occurred in the Nazi concentration camps (e.g., Dachau, Auschwitz, Buchenwald) and elsewhere, e.g., China, Japan, and, alas, the United States (e.g., untreated syphilitic patients at Tuskegee Institute in Alabama, 1932–72) were made known. The War Crimes Trial in Nuremberg (1946–7) surfaced the horrifying details of the actions of some prominent Nazi physicians who sought new medical knowledge to help their own soldiers but by means which were simply immoral. These revelations led to formulations or codes, such as the Nuremberg Code (NC) for medical experimentation, to protect the human subjects in medical experimentation. A number of other codes (such as the World Medical Association's 1964 Helsinki Declaration, revised at least three times since then) have been developed. These codes were in part a refinement of the NC and in part additions and changes in the light of new experience and new areas of research such as genetics, DNA, etc.

The Nuremberg Code set the stage for the subsequent codes which were developed for the purpose of protecting the human rights of human subjects of clinical research. The very first provision of the Code's ten provisions was: "The voluntary consent of the human subject is absolutely essential." To make sure that the intent, conditions, and content of that requirement was clearly understood, the code goes on to explain what it means:

> This means that the person involved should have the legal capacity to give consent; should be so situated as to be able to exercise free power of choice, without the intervention of any element of

force, fraud, deceit, duress, overreaching, or other ulterior form of constraint or coercion; and should have sufficient knowledge and comprehension of the elements of the subject matter involved as to enable him to make an understanding and enlightened decision. (George J. Annas and Michael A. Grodin, eds., *The Nazi Doctors and the Nuremberg Code* [New York: Oxford University Press, 1992], 121.

The obligation to see that this provision is properly fulfilled falls on the investigator and those who collaborate in the experiment:

> The duty and responsibility of ascertaining the quality of the consent rests upon each individual who initiates, directs or engages in the experiment. It is a personal duty and responsibility which may not be delegated to another with impunity. (Ibid.)

Thus, no one can later rightly claim that "I was just following orders." Each person involved is obliged to ascertain that proper free informed consent has been obtained from the human subjects of clinical research. In practice, however, it is not clear that all the participants have taken the time and trouble to verify that free informed consent was indeed obtained.

Catholic Teaching

From a Catholic perspective, human experimentation is not ruled out, but there are principles which are to be observed when carrying out research or experiments on human subjects. The address of Pope Pius XII to the First International Congress of Histopathology (September 13, 1952; Eng. trans., *The Human Body* [Boston: St. Paul Editions], #353–360, passim) well expresses the possibilities and the moral limitations of research with human subjects.

> For the moral justification of new processes, new experiments, and methods of research, three principles are invoked: 1) the interests of medical science; 2) the individual interests of the patient under treatment; 3) the common interests of the community, the "bonum commune".... Scientific knowledge has its own value in the domain of medical science ... a value which should by no means be minimized .... This does not mean, however, that every method ... becomes lawful by the fact that it increases and deepens our knowledge .... The doctor, as a private person, cannot take any measure or try any intervention without the consent of the patient. The doctor has only that power over the patient which the latter gives to him, be it explicitly, or implicitly and tacitly. The patient has not the right to involve his physical and psychic integrity in medical experiments or researches when these interventions entail, either immediately or subsequently, acts of destruction, or of mutilation and wounds, or grave dangers

Even more so, the protection of human dignity extends to subjects of human experimentation, that is, in particular for research which may not be therapeutic for the individual who is the subject of the research. Thus, there is a special Directive in the *Ethical and Religious Directives for Catholic Health Care Services* [1995]), on human research (#31):

> No one should be the subject of medical or genetic experimentation even if it is therapeutic, unless the person or surrogate first has given free and informed consent. In instances of nontherapeutic experimentation, the surrogate can give this consent only if the experiment entails no significant risk to the person's well-being. Moreover, the greater the person's incompetency and vulnerability, the greater the reasons must be to perform any medical experimentation, especially nontherapeutic.

Preserving Human Dignity

The Nazi medical war crimes were indeed atrocities. They helped the world realize that science, medical science, can be abused and that great care must be taken for the well-being of human subjects of medical research. As valuable as the knowledge may be in a particular situation, there is never any ethical warrant for the violation of the rights of any human subject, regardless of their age, medical condition, or their socioeconomic status.

What is at stake is the dignity of every human being, from conception until death. Medical experimentation with human subjects is indeed necessary and is good, but it must be carried out with a deep respect for the dignity and indeed the sacredness of every human being.

Rev. Albert S. Moraczewski, O.P., Ph.D., S.T.M.
President Emeritus
The National Catholic Bioethics Center
Boston, Massachusetts

Engaging the Public

Is The Written Law Ethical?

In a New York court opinion in 1811, the eminent Chancellor Kent asserted that "blasphemy is an offence [sic] ... at common law" which harms "the essential interests of society" and that the American people "profess the general doctrines of Christianity [sic]" (*The People against Ruggles,* 8 Johns 225). In one of the famous polygamy cases of the 1890s the U.S. Supreme Court stated: "Bigamy and polygamy are crimes by the laws of all civilized and Christian countries" and that "acts recognized by the general consent of the Christian world in modern times as proper matters for prohibitory legislation" can summon forth "the whole punitive power of government" (*Davis* v. *Beason*, 133 U.S. 333). The American courts of yesteryear, then, left little doubt that the transcendent moral law and Judeo-Christian moral principles could and should be embodied in our civil law.

Separating Morality from Law

Contrast this with more recent decisions of the U.S. Supreme Court. In the *Roe* v. *Wade* abortion opinion (410 U.S. 113), the Court forbade legislators from endorsing "one theory of life" and said it would not "speculate" as to when life begins. In its 1989 *Webster* v. *Reproductive Health Services* case, the Court upheld some limited state restrictions on abortion but did not say that government was obliged to protect innocent unborn human persons. In the 1990 case of *Cruzan* v. *Director, Missouri Department of Health,* the Court did not say that a debilitated person has an inherent right to the basic sustenance needed to continue life but just that the states may act in some circumstances to protect it. In other words, the Court has been unwilling to hold that the positive law must embody moral positions—even one so basic as the need to protect innocent human life—that are not the result of human consent. While some have interpreted *Webster* and *Cruzan* as moving in the direction of traditional Judeo-Christian belief, i.e., of the natural law, all the Court has really done is to give greater power to legislatures to act as they see fit in the areas in question. In short, it continues to be unwilling to ensconce sound ethics or, formally, *any* ethics into law.

This separation of law and ethics, in my judgment, has its immediate roots in such schools of legal philosophy as legal realism and sociological jurisprudence (predominant in the twentieth century), its intermediate roots in modern social science, and its distant roots in modern speculative philosophy.

Legal realism, usually associated with Justice Oliver Wendell Holmes, Jr., rejects the notion that there is a higher law discoverable by judges to use in adjudicating cases. Rather, it views law as simply *made* by judges. It is also emphatic about separating law from ethics. (See M. White, *Social Thought in America: The Revolt Against Formalism* [Boston: Beacon, 1957], 8, 65). Sociological jurisprudence teaches that the law "must be developed to keep up with social change"; its aim is to use law as an instrument of social reform (L. Lloyd of Hampstead, *Introduction to Jurisprudence* [New York: Praeger, 1960], 352). Neither perspective wanted to refer to a natural or transcendent moral law. Sociological jurisprudence was grounded upon positivistic assumptions and espouses social engineering. Holmes, the leading legal realist, advocated the "banish[ing]" of "every word of moral significance ... from the law" (quoted in White, *Social Thought*, 68).

Influence of Social Science

Contemporary theories of law have been considerably influenced by modern social science, especially the foundations as significantly shaped by Max Weber. In an attempt to make the study of society more scientific, Weber insisted upon the separation of facts and values. The social scientist, he argued, should study only phenomena; if he immersed himself in normative questions, e.g., questions of purpose and morality, he would thwart his objective of being scientific. This approach would not permit the neutrality Weber believed necessary. As Professor Leo Strauss puts it, Weber sought to avoid any "[r]eference to values" because this "presupposes appreciation of values." He did not want the social scientist to make judgments about which values are legitimate and which are not: there should be no endorsement of "ultimate values." Strauss concludes that Weber's thinking rested on the belief that "the conflict between ultimate values cannot be resolved by human reason" (L. Strauss, *Natural Right and History* [University of Chicago Press, 1953], 63–64).

Weber influenced legal thought as he did all the social sciences. The greatest impact he had on the "practical" side of law (e.g., on attitudes of judges on the judicial process) was probably with the notion that "ultimate values" or transcendent moral standards should not be allowed to shape the law. This norm of neutrality was, in fact, only capable of being carried into the realm of law and public policymaking to a limited degree. This is because it is not a practicable position for public decision makers, buffeted as they are by demands from groups and individual citizens. The latter do not want neutrality, they want their needs and wants met. Unwilling to turn to transcendent moral norms, judges, in response, have often made prevailing social theory their reference point even though it may or may not conform to true morality. *Roe* v. *Wade* is a case in point.

Denial of Universals

As stated, modern philosophy stands behind the above with its basic epistemological error. One writer describes it thus: "reality does [not] exist independently of the mind and ... can [not] be known with certainty" (J. Schmitt, "They No Longer Ask the Big Questions," in S. Krason, ed., *The Recovery of American Education* [Lanham, Md.: University. Press of America, 1991], 10–11). Having its origins in the medieval William of Occam, this is the position (in essence, the denial of universals) which is expressed in the conceptualism of Kant and his followers and by the nominalism of many modern thinkers. This denial of, or at least skepticism about, universals has logically led to a skepticism about universal moral norms. We live in a positivistic, relativistic era that doubts that morality can have any basis other than in human consent. In practice people often look to the civil law as their ethical reference point. I believe that we have witnessed this in American life with abortion. The curious point about this modern skepticism is that while it gained much of its force initially from the Renaissance and the Enlightenment, which glorified man's reason and believed it could carry him to unparalleled heights, it really has had the effect of debasing human reason. This is because it does not trust its ability to apprehend moral truth, or any reality.

The American Founding Tradition

In spite of the extent to which the ideas above have been imbibed by American law and other areas of our society, they do not represent our founding tradition. Noted political scientist Paul Eidelberg, for example, explains how the Declaration of Independence

> affirm[ed] ... the power of reason to apprehend transhistorical truths or the "laws of nature's God"... The appeal is from positive ... law to the natural/divine law ... [it] distinguishes between what is right by nature and what is right by convention, or between the just and the legal (P. Eidelberg, "Karl Marx and the Declaration of Independence: The Meaning of Marxism," in *The Intercollegiate Review,* 20:1, 4).

Eminent scholar Russell Kirk says our Founding Fathers appealed to a "natural law" tradition going back "to the principles of Cicero ... and the medieval schoolmen" (R. Kirk, *The Roots of American Order* [Malibu, CA: Pepperdine University Press, 1974], 403). Indeed, earlier Americans, a markedly religious people, did not question the validity of the moral norms of Christianity (i.e., the natural law). As Alexis deTocqueville said. "There is an innumerable multitude of sects in the United States ... [but] Christian morality is everywhere the same" (A. deTocqueville, *Democracy in America,* J.P. Mayer, ed., vol. 1 [Garden City, NY: Doubleday, 1966], 290–291).

The commitment to this genuine tradition of reason and to the natural law progressively weakened in American thought in the nineteenth century and affected the practical realms of our life in the twentieth century. To a large extent, this progressive weakening happened under the intensifying influence of secularization, although other factors were also involved. Thus, not only did our law fall prey to moral relativism, but so did our sexual ethics, medical ethics, and social ethics.

Eidelberg shows the substantial extent to which law and ethics were intertwined in the natural law tradition undergirding our founding. Not only could man know moral truth by his reason, but the validity of specific human laws was contingent on, at the very least, not being hostile to the natural law, whose content and viability are perennial and universal. Early in this tradition Aristotle argued that nature supplied standards of excellence, of right and wrong, and of virtue and vice. The Stoics advanced this tradition further by asserting that there was indeed a transcendent law, "right reason in accord with nature," which promulgates particular commands and prohibitions and originates in God. With St. Thomas Aquinas, the tradition advanced perhaps to its ultimate point. A clear hierarchy of law was developed with its origin in the divine intelligence; revelation is combined with the highest tradition of reason. In all these strains of the tradition, a transcendent standard of justice is used as the measure to evaluate the human law and the actions of regimes. As the great constitutional scholar Edward S. Corwin says, it is this very idea which underlay development of the American practice of judicial review (see E.S. Corwin, *The "Higher Law" Background of American Constitutional Law* [Ithaca, New York: Cornell University Press, 1955], 45).

Human Law and Ethics

Human law, of course, is not the same thing as ethics. While it must be based on sound ethical norms—on the natural law—it has a broader purpose. Its content may not, in some cases, directly reflect or pertain to the natural law. Many parts of the civil law are indeed declarative of the natural law, i.e., they represent an implementing of the precepts of natural law into positive law. Other parts, however, that are needed for the sake of good order may be enacted by human lawgivers but involve matters which are morally neutral. Our problem today, as mentioned above, is that we sometimes treat human law as if it is ethics, that is, as if it designates what is morally right. This reflects the belief that both law and morals are derived from little more than human consent or opinion; this is moral relativism. Thus we often see conflict between law and medical ethics nowaday. To avoid these conflicts, I believe that American society needs to return to the tradition from which it emerged: the tradition of the natural law.

Stephen M. Krason, J.D., Ph.D.
Professor of Political Science
Franciscan University of Steubenville
Steubenville, Ohio
President, Society of Catholic Social Scientists

Catholic Hospitals and Abortion Physicians

Central to the Catholic hospital's identity, meaning, and mission is its commitment to the teaching of the Catholic Church on the dignity of human life, which must be respected from the moment of conception through natural death. As witness to that commitment, the Catholic health care institution has taken a firm and unwavering stand against direct abortion. Though many have challenged the institution's "right" to disallow such abortions, that right has been upheld consistently in the courts (*Doe* v. *Bellin Memorial Hospital* [May 1973]; *Watkins* v. *Mercy Medical Center* [July 1973]; Health Programs Extension Act of 1973). Those laws which seek to protect decisions of conscience apply equally to institutions and to individuals.

However, the same laws which allow the Catholic institution to exercise this right threaten its ability to maintain a clear and consistent witness in this regard. What enables the Catholic institution to refuse to provide abortion services also ensures that persons associated with (or wishing to be associated with) the institution may not be barred on the basis of their actions outside of the institution (Patricia Younger, ed., *Hospital Law Manual* [Rockville, MD: Aspen Publications], 44).

Thus, according to the law, while a physician on the staff of a Catholic hospital may be constrained from performing a direct abortion within the Catholic institution, that physician cannot be removed from the staff because he performs abortions elsewhere. Neither can a physician applying for privileges be denied admission to the medical staff on the grounds that he participates in abortions elsewhere.

The problem raised for the Catholic health care institution is this: granting of staff privileges to a physician implies approval of that physician and his practice. If privileges are extended to a physician who participates in abortions elsewhere, how is the Catholic hospital to maintain a clear and unambiguous witness to the value of human life, especially when staff privileges provides the physician with a source of patients, income, and the opportunity to practice and perfect his art?

One Solution to the Problem

Generally, these kinds of questions are answered by appeal to the principle of legitimate cooperation. Thus, an argument seeking to explain the presence of physicians on a Catholic hospital's medical staff who perform abortions elsewhere might be structured as follows.

In carrying out its ministry, the Catholic hospital may choose to offer obstetric and gynecologic services in a manner consistent with the teaching of the Catholic Church. But in order to do so the hospital must have an adequate number of physicians on its medical staff who are qualified in these areas.

Not all physicians agree with Catholic belief and teaching, and the law prohibits the Catholic institution from denying privileges to physicians based on their agreement or disagreement with Catholic belief and teaching. Therefore, the Catholic hospital may be forced to extend staff privileges to a physician who requests such a position but who also performs abortions elsewhere. In gaining access to the medical staff, the physician necessarily is allowed the use of the hospital's facilities, as well as allowed access to various resources and benefits from association with the Catholic hospital.

However, in granting these privileges, the Catholic institution *does not cooperate formally* with the physician in the performance of morally illicit practices at other institutions. Rather, the cooperation forced on the Catholic institution by the law in such circumstances is *material cooperation:* the Catholic hospital *neither intends nor approves of the evil* which the physician does in performing an abortion elsewhere but intends only the good of providing needed services in the Catholic context (Ashley and O'Rourke, *Health Care Ethics: A Theological Analysis,* 4th ed. [Washington, D.C.: Georgetown University Press, 1997], 193–197).

The fact that the Catholic institution *would not grant staff privileges to such physicians were it not compelled to do so by the law* further indicates that the cooperation is *material.* The Catholic institution's only aim is to provide obstetric and gynecologic services to the community. The good of providing these services in a Catholic context outweighs the presence on the medical staff of a physician who participates in morally illicit procedures elsewhere.

Is it sufficient, however, simply to offer an explanation of the principle of material cooperation where the Catholic institution, because of legal constraints, must grant staff privileges to requesting physicians who perform abortions elsewhere?

Because the Catholic hospital's commitment to respect and support human life is integral to its identity as *Catholic,* the answer must be "no." In order to reaffirm this commitment and address the potential scandal that may be caused by the presence of such physicians on the Catholic institution's medical staff, it is necessary to establish that the form of material cooperation involved is *remote* rather than proximate.

Appropriate Measures

Let me propose, then, a series of steps that the Catholic hospital should take *in addition to* providing a clear explanation of the principle of material cooperation to insure that such cooperation is remote.

The assumption underlying my proposal is this: The Catholic hospital is an integral part of the mission and ministry of Jesus and the Church. As such, it is accountable to the broader Christian community and has an obligation to educate that community with regard to all issues affecting its ability to carry out its mission. At the same time, it is important that the ordinary of the diocese be consulted and involved prior to the beginning of negotiations with any non-Catholic party associated with practices at variance with Catholic moral teaching.

Explaining Remote Cooperation

What, then, should the Catholic hospital do when, in accordance with the law, it may not turn away physicians requesting staff privileges *solely* on the grounds that the physician engages in an illicit procedure elsewhere?

First, the hospital should ascertain the extent of the physician's involvement in abortion activities. It is one thing if participation in abortions occurred during a residency program or at some time in the past. It is quite another if the physician is currently involved in providing direct abortions. Further complications would arise if the physician operated an "abortion clinic" in the same community where the Catholic hospital is located.

Second, the hospital should establish a process for *on-going* dialogue between the physician(s), hospital administration, and other appropriate persons, by which the position of the Catholic institution with regard to direct abortion can be clearly stated and reaffirmed. It should be made clear to the physician that, while the Catholic hospital grants him medical staff privileges, it does so unwillingly.

Third, openly educate the community which the Catholic hospital serves as to the nature of the dilemma facing the institution. Make it known that the law does not allow the Catholic institution to limit medical staff privileges only to those physicians who agree in word and deed with Catholic beliefs and values. Emphasize that, in complying with the law by granting staff privileges to a physician who requests them and who performs abortions elsewhere, the Catholic hospital does not, thereby, approve of the physician's behavior. Were it possible, the hospital *would not* grant privileges to such physicians.

Finally, if necessary, raise the hard questions. For example, does the presence of such physicians on the Catholic hospital's staff so undermine the institution's credibility and witness that some thought should be given to discontinuing obstetric and gynecologic services? Answers will depend, of course, on how many physicians on the staff are involved in abortion procedures elsewhere, the extent of their involvement, their visibility in the community, and whether other nearby Catholic facilities are providing similar procedures. A decision to discontinue these obstetric and gynecological services in a Catholic hospital should be necessary only in extreme circumstances.

With Reluctance Only

Addressing these issues openly will not make them any easier to deal with. It will, however, clearly show that the Catholic hospital *reluctantly* admits physicians who request staff privileges and who perform abortions elsewhere because of legal constraints against discrimination in hiring because of behavior inconsistent with Catholic beliefs. That is, it will show that the Catholic institution's cooperation in these circumstances is both *material* and *remote.*

Sr. Jean DeBlois, C.S.J., Ph.D.
Vice President, Mission Services
Catholic Health Association
St. Louis, Missouri

Individual and Corporate Cooperation

The impressive realism and coherence of Christian morality is based in part upon the fundamental convictions that 1) there is an objective moral order which can be known by the intellect and that 2) some actions are "intrinsically evil," that is, they are never morally justifiable regardless of the circumstances of the act. This is one of the major teachings of *Veritatis splendor*. Three theological principles have been developed to deal with the ethical permissibility of actions which relate to either physical evil or the moral evil of other agents. These are known as 1) the principle of the double effect (see article in this volume); 2) the choice of the "lesser evil"; and 3) the principles of cooperation. These concepts have been taught and reflected upon, and, with the exception of the second (lesser evil), they have enjoyed generally unquestioned acceptance in philosophical ethics and Catholic moral theology.

Historical Origins

St. Alphonsus Liguori (d. 1787) made the principles of cooperation acceptable by introducing the distinction between formal and material cooperation and by a consideration of scandal as a serious invitation to sin. Cooperation in the ethically significant sense is defined as the participation of one agent in the activity of another agent to produce a particular effect or share in a joint activity. This becomes ethically problematical when the action of the primary agent is morally wrong.

There are three basic examples of cooperation on the part of individuals: the cooperation of the hostage, of the taxpayer, and of the accomplice. The participation or cooperation of these individuals in morally questionable acts of the principal agent is quite distinct one from another. The hostage is forced with threats to comply with the evil act of another person. Fear more or less compels the hostage to cooperate. This diminishes his culpability and in some cases eliminates it completely. In contrast, the accomplice may perform the same act as the hostage, but culpability is imputed fully because cooperation in this instance is free and willed (directly intended). The taxpayer is an example of one who cooperates with a principal agent (the government) in an important—in fact, essential—mission (societal governance). Nevertheless, it is possible that the government may sponsor activities which are immoral. The taxpayer then contributes in some degree to this immoral activity. However, contributing to the stability of society is not an intrinsic evil but a good.

The Principal Distinctions

Among the principles of cooperation, the primary distinction is between formal and material cooperation. Formal cooperation is a willing participation on the part of the cooperative agent in the sinful act of the principal agent. This formal cooperation can either be explicit ("Yes, I'm happy to drive the getaway car because I want to be an accomplice") or implicit. "Implicit formal cooperation is attributed when, even though the cooperator denies intending the wrongdoer's object, no other explanation can distinguish the cooperator's object from the wrongdoer's object" (*Ethical and Religious Directives for Catholic Health Services* [1995], Appendix). The motto of the implicit formal cooperator is "I am personally opposed, but ..." This cooperation is as immoral as explicit formal cooperation.

Material cooperation has several inherent distinctions, the most basic is that between immediate and mediate material cooperation. Theologians maintain that in the objective order, immediate material cooperation is equivalent to implicit formal cooperation because the object of the moral act of the cooperator is indistinguishable from that of the principal agent. Those who use the term "immediate material cooperation" have understood this as ethically unacceptable behavior when the principal agent's act is intrinsically evil. An example of this would be any form of employment in an abortion clinic.

Immediate material cooperation is contrasted with mediate cooperation. Here the moral object of the cooperator's act is not that of the wrongdoer's. (An example of this would be a health care worker employed in a secular hospital that also provides for morally prohibited procedures, but does not require the conscientious objector to such procedures to participate.) This kind of cooperation can be justified 1) for a sufficient reason and 2) if scandal can be avoided. It is a form of cooperating with the circumstances surrounding the wrongdoer's act. Depending on how closely these circumstances impinge upon the act, there is a distinction between proximate and remote material cooperation. (Proximate material cooperation would be, for example, the work of the recovery room nurse who cares for all post-surgical patients, including those who may have undergone morally illicit procedures. This form of routine care is not intrinsically evil.)

Further, necessary material cooperation is that without which the sinful act could not occur. Contingent cooperation (also called free cooperation) is that without which the evil act would still take place. An example of necessary material cooperation would be cooperating if one is the only anesthesiologist available to assist with a woman undergoing a combination C-section and tubal ligation. Contingent material cooperation would exist if one were not the only such professional available.

Application to Corporate Partnerships

The theological development of the principles of cooperation has considered the actions of *individuals* who cooperate with the evil actions of others. Contemporary theological considerations are not so restricted. There are questions about "corporate actions" of cooperation, such as joint ventures between health care institutions which may be morally questionable because some actions of one of the partner institutions may be ethically unacceptable to the other cooperative institution.

Very few acts of the non-Catholic partner may be morally wrong, and the rest quite good. Apart from the morally illicit procedures, their provision of health care is not intrinsically evil. That is why the analogy of the taxpayer to describe this cooperation is so apt.

A complicating factor here is the fact that "cooperation" between institutions or systems is an arrangement made on the level of a legal corporation. The cooperative venture has a very precise and clearly defined identity and purpose, which may not be evident in public discussion. The partnership is a legal and/or corporate structuring intended to perform only functions

1) which are mutually agreeable to all partners;

2) which do not include any procedures which any partner disagrees with on moral grounds; and

3) which explicitly separate the partnership for activities not approved by all partners, which an individual partner may continue to engage in.

Why is this sort of partnering necessary? There are several reasons. First, clinical medicine has reduced the need for the present number of hospital beds. Many procedures are handled on an outpatient basis, more complicated procedures require a shorter hospital recovery period, and, in the health care market, competition is a cost-driving, not a cost-containing force. The need to downsize acute care settings and to create state-of-the-art diagnostic and day treatment centers has led to the realization that health care delivery must be reorganized in more efficient forms, which is often referred to as "rationalizing" care.

The practical conclusion to this reconfiguration is that a "stand-alone" position is not always a viable option. In most cases, it is foreseen that isolation would entail eventual closure. Market pressure is considered a "sufficient reason," which is one of the "ingredients" necessary to justify material cooperation.

Scandal must also be overcome. Scandal is not the same as a public relations problem. Scandal is the serious suggestion that evil is attractive or permissible. Any partnering between Catholic and non-Catholic health services must avoid the impression that Catholic moral doctrine is not being observed.

Five Basic Principles

The National Catholic Bioethics Center uses five basic principles to evaluate partnerships: 1) Cooperation must be mediate material, never formal nor immediate material; 2) We can only do together what all partners agree to be appropriate, so while the partnership need not be Catholic, it must nevertheless observe the *Ethical and Religious Directives* as respecting the "corporate conscience" of the Catholic partner; 3) Morally illicit procedures cannot be provided on the Catholic campus; 4) Any morally illicit procedure(s) provided on campuses of non-Catholic alliance partners must be excluded from the new alliance corporation through separate incorporation (governance, administration, and finance); and 5) All publicity should be straightforward, i.e., the need to form an alliance for the survival of a worthy apostolate should be made known; the good achieved by rationalizing health care must be to the patients' benefit; immoral procedures must be excluded from the partnership (while these services may still be available on the campuses of some partner[s]). This publicity should also appear in the promotional literature of the Catholic hospital. The observance of these principles should issue in a morally sound and scandal-free partnership that will contribute to the Catholic health care tradition.

Rev. Russell E. Smith, S.T.D.
Theological and Health Care Consultant
Diocese of Richmond, Virginia

Growth in the Market

Avoiding Formal Cooperation in Health Care Alliances

Replacement of traditional fee-for-service health care with capitation, the rising costs of new medical technologies, the duplication of health services among competitors, and the need to attract physician networks and managed care contracts are some of the factors that necessitate collaborative efforts among health care facilities. Although the *Ethical and Religious Directives for Health Care Services* [1995] state that Catholic facilities should seek alliances with other Catholic institutions first, unfortunately, it is not always possible to find them.

When a potential local collaborator is engaging in procedures that contradict Catholic moral teaching by violating the dignity of human persons, the Catholic teaching on the principles of cooperation comes into play. The operative directive here is #69, which states:

> When a Catholic health care institution is participating in a partnership that may be involved in activities judged morally wrong by the Church, the Catholic institution should limit its involvement in accord with the moral principles governing cooperation.

This directive states that Catholic institutions should use the principles of cooperation in order to limit involvement in evil with non-Catholic providers, not expand it. However, cooperation is the moral principle which is used to discern permissible types of collaboration with those doing evil, and we at the Center attempt to use it as far as possible.

The aim of this article is to set forth, in as clear a manner as possible, how The National Catholic Bioethics Center uses the principles of cooperation to assess whether or not a given collaborative venture between Catholic and non-Catholic health care institutions crosses the line into Catholic moral culpability for the evil which is being perpetrated in the non-Catholic institution.

Directive #69 is the only directive which refers to "the moral principles governing cooperation." The *Directives* then provide a brief explanation of the principles of cooperation in an Appendix. However, it should be remembered that the Appendix is but a brief explanation of the principles and is not as useful as a fuller exposition would have been. In the Preamble to the *Direc-*

tives, the bishops do say that this document will have to be revised from time to time, and we believe that the Appendix could certainly be modified on some points in the future. Nonetheless, it does serve as a point of departure for those providing a moral analysis of proposed collaborative ventures between Catholic institutions and non-Catholic institutions that may be involved in evil.

At the outset, we state that we understand *cooperation* (*in moral evil*) *to be the free and knowing assistance of an individual in an immoral act, either as a means or an end, principally performed by another person* (*the principal agent*).

The Appendix to the *Directives* states that the principles of cooperation differentiate the action of the wrongdoer from the action of the cooperator. Two important points of clarification can be made about this starting point in order to understand the purposes of the principles of cooperation. First, the cooperator is obviously not immune from becoming a wrongdoer. Some types of cooperation cross the line into the actual doing of evil so that there are two wrongdoers: the original wrongdoer and the cooperator. The principles of cooperation presume that we know the different kinds of wrongdoing. What needs articulation are the different sorts of cooperation which can serve as a guide for the cooperator to avoid evil while doing and pursuing good.

It should be obvious that there is never any other motivation for the Catholic institution to consider cooperating with those who may be engaged in certain immoral activities than to pursue good, which in this case is the provision of health care to those in need, particularly to those least able to obtain it. However, we cannot pretend that there is not a cultural context within which Catholics must make their judgment with respect to a given instance of cooperation, and the dominant culture is simply no longer repulsed by acts which, until recently, were universally viewed as morally repugnant such as abortion, euthanasia, physician-assisted suicide, indeed even contraception.

Formal and Material Cooperation

The Appendix first divides cooperation into its two well-known types, formal and material, and states "If the cooperator intends the object of the wrongdoer's activity, then the cooperation is formal and, therefore, morally wrong." The "moral object" is the kind of act performed. Thus, if two people intend to procure an abortion and work together to procure the abortion, they share the same moral object.

However, while we do not disagree with that definition, it may be too narrowly worded to account for the full dimension of formal cooperation. The morality of the cooperator's act or of the principal agent's act is determined in either case not only by 1) the "moral object" or kind of action performed, but also by 2) the intention with which the act is performed and 3) the circumstances associated with the act (the traditional "fonts" of morality). The cooperator can participate in different ways in any of these three components of the principal agent's act. The Appendix correctly, but we believe incompletely, defines formal cooperation only in terms of the *object* of the principal agent's act. When the Center evaluates a collaborative venture, actual or proposed, *we understand formal cooperation to be the intending or concurring in any one or more of the immoral components of the principal agent's act, either as an end in itself or as a means.* One could intend an essential circumstance for the commission of an evil without directly intending the evil itself. One could, for example, intentionally provide some of the circumstances necessary for the performance of an abortion without actually willing the abortion.

Implicit Formal Cooperation Not Permitted

According to the Appendix, "Implicit formal cooperation is attributed when, even though the cooperator denies intending the wrongdoer's object, no other explanation can distinguish the cooperator's object from the wrongdoer's object." Also it should be noted that although Directive #69 states that the involvement of the Catholic institution with those doing evil should be limited by the moral principles governing cooperation, the directive does not state that they are necessarily or fully applicable to collaborative ventures between Catholic and non-Catholic institutions. Based upon our definition of formal cooperation given above, *we understand implicit formal cooperation to be intending any one or more of the immoral components of the principal agent's act but as a means to something other than the principal agent's act.* In our judgment Catholic health care institutions are especially susceptible to implicit formal cooperation.

For example, a Catholic hospital may explicitly reject the immoral activities of a potential non-Catholic partner and yet forge a legally binding agreement by means of which the non-Catholic partner is able to continue to engage in the immoral practices, which simply come to be performed someplace else. But the physical distance of the immoral practices from the Catholic hospital is morally irrelevant if the Catholic institution is contractually committed to enabling the non-Catholic institution to continue the immoral practices through the provision of such things as space, personnel, surgical instruments, and financing. When such collaboration occurs it is invariably provided by the Catholic institution not to bring about the immoral procedures, to be sure, but to seek other ends such as financial stability or the continuing provision of health care to the poor. Nonetheless, the immoral procedures would not be taking place but for the collaboration of the Catholic hospital. We would view such involvement as implicit formal cooperation.

Therefore, as applied to health care collaboration agreements, implicit formal cooperation would include such things as the negotiating, writing, or consenting to agreements which establish the governance, management, or financing of the immoral procedures of another health care entity, or any institutional participation in those procedures and activities. Implicit and explicit formal cooperation are both wrong under any circumstances and both are rejected by the *Ethical and Religious Directives*.

Material Cooperation, Licit and Illicit

Licit Material Cooperation (*Mediate*)

With respect to material cooperation, the Appendix states, "If the cooperator does not intend the object of the wrongdoer's activity, the cooperation is material and *can be* morally licit." [Emphasis added.] This definition does not account for another characteristic of material cooperation which distinguishes it from formal cooperation, namely, that the cooperator contributes only to the circumstances of the principal agent's act. *When the cooperator contributes only to the morally licit circumstances associated with the principal agent's act, and those circumstances are not essential to the principal agent's performance of the evil action, we can say that the cooperation is mediate material and may be morally licit.*

The Appendix states that material cooperation should be "as distant as possible" from the wrongdoer's act. The term "distant" in the context of collaborative arrangements is often wrongly interpreted to mean a geographic distance, or a distance in the number of levels of management that the Catholic hospital is removed from the immoral procedures. However, even if a distance in these senses is achieved, Catholic health care institutions can still engage in immoral cooperation through their operating agreements. Instead of using the word "distant," it should be said that the more an institution is causally removed from the immoral procedure or activity, the more acceptable is its material cooperation.

Illicit Material Cooperation (*Immediate*)

The Appendix states that the "material cooperation is immediate when the object of the cooperator is the same as the object of the wrongdoer." Here the language of the Appendix lacks a certain clarity. For if the cooperator shares the same object as the wrongdoer, then as the Appendix itself stated earlier with respect to formal cooperation, "the cooperator intends the object of the wrongdoer's activity." Thus in the Appendix the terms "formal cooperation" and "immediate material cooperation" share the same meaning, and we may substitute the one for the other whenever either occurs.

The Appendix then goes on to state that "immediate material cooperation is wrong, except in some instances of duress." Let us, at this point, perform the substitution. If we substitute "formal cooperation" for "immediate material cooperation" in the preceding sentence, we arrive at "formal cooperation is wrong, except in some instances of duress." When duress is not present, immediate material cooperation, in the words of the Appendix, "is equivalent to implicit formal cooperation and, therefore, is morally wrong." Thus it would seem that it is possible to read the Appendix as justifying some instances of formal cooperation in intrinsically immoral acts if these occur under duress. However, this cannot be what the Appendix means to say. Clearly there is a need for greater clarity in explaining these differences.

In our view, material cooperation arises when the cooperator does not intend the object of the principal agent's act, but nonetheless contributes to the circumstances surrounding that act. If the circumstances are not essential to the carrying out of the wrongful act, the cooperation is mediate material and may be licit depending upon the gravity of the moral object of the wrongdoer and the question of scandal. Immediate material cooperation, in our view, is the contribution of the cooperator to circumstances that are essential to the commission of the principal agent's immoral act and is not licit.

Immediate Material Cooperation and Duress

One problem with the explanation of immediate material cooperation in the Appendix is that duress is not defined. In our view, immediate material cooperation remains immoral because most instances of duress do not change the fact that the cooperator voluntarily contributes to circumstances that are essential to the principal agent's act. The cooperator may indeed act through fear of the loss of some great good, but this fear does not force the will, since the will cannot act under compulsion (see Thomas Aquinas, *Summa Theologiae* I-II, 6.4–6). However, the fear that results from duress is a circumstance that substantially alters the culpability of the cooperator, diminishing it or eliminating it altogether.

The Center understands immediate material cooperation as any willful, intentional contribution to the circumstances essential to the principal agent's immoral act. Considered in itself, immediate material cooperation in evil is wrong, but its culpability is significantly reduced or eliminated if done through a legitimate fear of losing a great good.

As has been often noted, the principles of cooperation were originally formulated to assess the morality of cooperative actions of individuals. On an institutional level those who defend cooperating with a wrongdoer in an immediately material manner through some collaborative arrangement on the grounds of duress employ arguments that require us to transfer their reasoning from individuals to corporations. This simply does not always work. One of the major areas of difficulty concerns the question of whether any potential harm that might face a corporate person could be equivalent to that possibly faced by an individual person

Consider the following example. A clerk held at gunpoint is told to open the store safe. If he refuses to do so, he has reason to believe he will be killed. When the clerk agrees to open the safe, he consents to what appears to be immediate material cooperation in evil, for he agrees to participate directly in the commission of the crime of theft and his actions contribute in an essential way to that act. There are several ways in which the act of the clerk might be justified. For example, because the good of life is preferable to the good of property, this decision is justified by the choice of life over property. Or it might be questioned whether this was even truly an act of cooperation, since we had defined cooperation earlier as the voluntary participation of one individual in the act of another. In this case, the threat of the loss of life and the accompanying fear could so reduce the free exercise of the will that one might question whether the act can even properly be evaluated in terms of the principles of cooperation.

However, in our opinion, neither line of reasoning is applicable to a health care institution or corporate person. No human life is in jeopardy or under threat when a Catholic hospital closes down or is sold to a non-Catholic buyer, as regrettable and as tragic as that may be. There could be diminished access to quality health care in a given community, but this is not a Catholic problem as such nor one for which the Catholic entity would be morally culpable. The problem of lack of access to adequate health care is a profound social concern in our day beyond the capability of all of Catholic health care to resolve. It is true that the financial health and perhaps even the life of the Catholic institution may be at stake, but the loss of a Catholic health care facility is simply not equivalent to the loss of the life of a human being. This is one reason why it is difficult to apply the principles of cooperation and/or duress to corporate persons.

There is another reason why the principles of cooperation do not easily apply to institutions. The fact of the matter is that Catholic institutions are bound to a more rigorous application of the principles limiting cooperation in evil than are individuals, because Catholic institutions stand as very public witnesses to Catholic teaching and morality. The Holy Father, John Paul II, repeatedly speaks of the necessity of reevangelizing culture, and the public witness of Catholic institutions to Catholic morality can serve as tremendous impetus for positive social change and the attainment of greater social justice because the very foundation of Catholic morality is commitment to the dignity and integrity of the human person.

We must remember that the fundamental purpose of any Catholic apostolate is to bear witness to Jesus Christ and the salvation which He won for all. Jesus cured the man crippled from birth, not primarily to allow him to walk, but primarily to provide proof that He, Jesus of Nazareth, had the power to forgive sins, a power reserved to God Himself. Jesus healed physically in order to give witness to a greater healing which He and his Church offer, healing from moral evil. Catholic institutions can do nothing which would contribute to the advancement of evil in the world, nor can they do anything which would lead to confusion in people's minds about what constitutes sin without betraying Jesus Christ Himself, in other words, without betraying the One who gives meaning to their very existence. Sacrifice of moral principle for the sake of financial gain, for the sake of an increase in market share, for the sake of gaining a competitive edge, even for the sake of serving the poor cannot be legitimate, for Catholic institutions must give constant preference to spiritual goods over those that are temporal.

Institutionalized Cooperation

Another serious difficulty in trying to apply the notion of duress to corporate persons concerns institutionalizing a kind of cooperation which may be legitimate on a one-time basis but not on a continuing basis. It would be strange indeed if the clerk who opened the safe to save his life continued to collaborate with the robber even after the threat of force was over, but this is exactly what sometimes happens to a Catholic health care facility when it agrees, because of "duress," to immediate material cooperation in the provision of contraceptive sterilization, for example, or any other intrinsically immoral act. After the questionable collaborative arrangement is signed—and the potential financial or other disaster has been averted—the Catholic partner finds itself contractually committed to continued cooperation in immoral procedures.

Thus the duress that was originally used to justify cooperation has passed, but the "immediate material cooperation" in evil has not. Such institutional cooperation in non-death-dealing immoral acts might be possible on a one-time or even an episodic basis (for example, if a court injunction should order a Catholic hospital to allow the performance of a direct surgical sterilization), but it cannot become an integral part of the daily, ongoing operations of the Catholic facility. We hold that when a Catholic health care facility makes an institutional commitment to facilitating immoral practices by another institution with which it is collaborating, it engages in implicit formal cooperation. When parties sign their names to an operating agreement, they express their intention to carry out certain actions jointly or to exclude certain activities from their joint actions. Whatever the parties agree to do in writing constitute the elements on which they formally agree to cooperate, or they identify those areas in which they will not cooperate in order to achieve their common goals.

While contraceptive sterilizations and abortions may constitute the most common obstacles to collaboration with many non-Catholic health care institutions today, it must be remembered that the number of morally repugnant activities which are becoming increasingly culturally accepted continues to grow. Catholic hospitals must be prepared to avoid culpable involvement also in other immoral procedures, such as *in vitro* fertilization, artificial insemination by spouse or donor, the use of donor eggs, the cryo-preservation of embryos, fetal experimentation, physician-assisted suicide, and euthanasia. As stated previously, when an operating agreement states that the Catholic partner will not engage in certain immoral procedures, but that the Catholic agent nonetheless will assist the non-Catholic partner in setting up a new facility or in making use of an existing facility or personnel or equipment for the performance of these same procedures, this must be viewed as implicit formal cooperation. Despite the claims of the Catholic hospital, the enabling clauses of the operating agreement clearly show that the immoral procedures come into being, or continue in existence, only through the collaborating agency of the Catholic partner.

The Terms of the Operating Agreement

Collaborative arrangements with a non-Catholic entity that wishes to engage in immoral activities must require that the non-Catholic agent carry out the procedures entirely through its own agency and on its own premises, and that it be the sole cause of any facility or practice which is established specifically for their provision. The operating agreement may acknowledge the kinds of activities in which the non-Catholic institution will be engaged and to which the Catholic entity will not be party because of its moral convictions, but the agreement cannot have the effect of making the Catholic partner assist in the provision of the immoral procedures or practices.

The collaborative agreement should also specify the activities in which the Catholic entity will not be engaged; for example, it should not simply refer to "prohibited or proscribed activities" but rather to specific activities such as *in vitro* fertilization or the freezing of embryos or surrogate mothering or physician-assisted suicide. In addition to the specification of those acts which Catholics believe do violence to the dignity of the human person, the agreement should also note that the Catholic hospital will not involve itself in procedures which the Magisterium of the Church would in the future judge to be immoral. It should note that the local ordinary should act as the final arbiter on such matters and as the ultimate interpreter of the *Ethical and Religious Directives* and their application within his jurisdiction.

This article reflects our current understanding of the way in which the principles of cooperation can best be used to deal with collaboration between Catholic and non-Catholic health care institutions. It demonstrates the manner in which we use them in the cases of collaboration which are submitted to us. We invite other Catholic ethicists to offer comments on and criticisms of our views, with the hope that within the Church a more consistent approach can be found to assess the morality of collaborative arrangements so that the Catholic health care apostolate can be strengthened in its contemporary mission of serving those in need, in imitation of Christ.

The Ethicists
The National Catholic Bioethics Center
Boston, Massachusetts

Models of Collaborative Arrangements

Presuming the approach explained in the preceding chapter, I will outline some models of collaboration that the NCBC has found to be conducive to licit cooperation and others that, in our opinion, commit the Catholic institution to implicit formal cooperation.

Cooperation and Collaboration

The initial efforts at constructing collaboration proposals are significantly aided by a *prima facie* principle for evaluating the risk of immoral cooperation: The risk of immoral cooperation in a health care collaboration is proportionate to the level of institutional integration present in the collaboration. Consequently, the greater the integration, the greater the risk of unacceptable cooperation in what Catholic moral teaching regards as morally objectionable procedures. Consistent with this principle, the analysis will proceed by examining collaboration models with minimal institutional integration (Limited Affiliations), and move to a model with maximum institutional integration (Joint Operating Company). It is important to note that while these models are conducive to morally acceptable cooperation they cannot by themselves legitimate any particular collaboration arrangement, nor do they necessarily overcome possible scandal.

Models of Licit Collaboration

Each Limited Affiliation model includes these essential characteristics: 1) there is no institutional integration of governance, management, or finances; 2) there are certain reserved powers critical to the preservation of institutional independence; 3) each institution retains its own assets and liabilities; 4) any and all joint activities must be in compliance with the *Ethical and Religious Directives for Catholic Health Care Services*, or with a morally equivalent "Common Values Statement" that prohibits specific procedures. This fourth common characteristic is established by a "mission" or "values" section in the joint agreement. It is also secured by sections in the agreement that provide for conflict resolution and exit strategies that both preserve the business purposes of the affiliation and protect the Catholic partner from illicit cooperation. To avoid scandal, the non-Catholic partner to the arrangement must agree not to provide abortion.

Joint Venture Agreement: Two health care institutions jointly operate or provide one or a limited number of functions or services. For example, hospital A and hospital B might jointly operate pathology services.

Master Affiliation Agreement (MAA): Two or more health care institutions enter into an agreement that creates a "Preferred Status" between the affiliates for collaboration on a range of services and functions. Examples of what could be included are: Behavioral Health; Extended Care; Ambulatory Care; Physician Networks; Rehabilitation Services; Managed Care Contracting; Academic Affiliation; Acute Care Services; Clinical Laboratories; Diagnostic Services; and Administrative and Support Services. (These examples also apply to the LMC and the JMC below.) The MAA includes provisions that exclude the same relationships with non-affiliating institutions and identifies existing and potential geographical areas and organizations for possible affiliations. The agreement also stipulates that the terms and conditions for collaborative arrangements on individual services will be set forth in "Separate Agreements" that comply with the MAA. Management of individual collaborative arrangements is not provided by a joint company but by the institutions that have established a Separate Agreement.

Limited Management Company (LMC): The purpose of an LMC is to facilitate joint ventures between the collaborating institutions. The LMC Operating Agreement provides for a Board of Managers that is responsible for: 1) strategic planning; 2) program development for joint ventures; 3) a business plan; and 4) an annual budget. The Operating Agreement also establishes rights of first refusal and rights of participation in new transactions of the collaborating institutions. The joint venture participants capitalize, own, operate, and manage the joint ventures apart from the LMC.

Joint Management Company (JMC): The Operating Agreement of the JMC provides for a Board with the same responsibilities as those for an LMC. The essential difference between an LMC and a JMC is that the JMC has the added function of actually managing and being a profit center for the joint ventures.

The Limited Affiliation models carry little to no risk of formal cooperation in the morally objectionable procedures of a non-Catholic partner as long as their corporate structures retain the four characteristics mentioned above. The models do not present any mechanism (either governance, management, or financing) by which the morally objectionable procedures of a non-Catholic partner are made possible. The only collaboration between the institutions is for specific joint ventures and programs that must comply with the *Directives*, or a morally equivalent "Common Values Statement." This fact leaves only licit material cooperation (if any at all), because the collaboration either does not, or only remotely, contributes to circumstances associated with the procedures in question.

Joint Operating Company (JOC): The purpose of a JOC is to create a centralized management authority over the collaborating institutions which otherwise retain their independence in some important ways, e.g., separate governance, identities, assets and liabilities, and medical staffs. The scope of the JOC's authority extends from day-to-day operations of the system, to managed care contracting, to approval of capital expenditures. The high level of management integration between the collaborating institutions creates an increased risk of formal cooperation in any morally objectionable procedures provided by the non-Catholic partner. If the non-Catholic partner provides morally objectionable procedures, their governance, management, and financing must be completely segregated from the JOC. This segregation cannot be established through the Joint Operating Agreement, or by any representatives of the Catholic partner, although the fact of who will provide the procedures can be recognized in the agreement. As with the Limited Affiliation models, the JOC activities must comply with the *ERD*s, or a morally equivalent "Common Values Statement."

Merger and Consolidation: Mergers and consolidations are not collaborations but they can radically affect the identity of a Catholic health care institution. In a merger one hospital is subsumed into another "surviving corporation" that retains its identity. In a health care consolidation two or more entities join and lose their corporate identities to a new corporation. A consolidation or a merger has a single corporate identity. This fact means that what each member institution does, it does in the name of the whole system. Therefore, each member must comply with the *Directives* or a morally equivalent "Common Values Statement" in order for a consolidation or a merger to fulfill its Catholic identity. If in the case of a merger the removal of the procedures from the non-Catholic facility must be delayed for financial or logistical reasons, the assets of the non-Catholic hospital can be acquired by a nonprofit community based group on a temporary basis with certain powers being reserved to the Catholic institution so that control and ownership can be transferred to the Catholic institution once the morally objectionable procedures are removed.

Models of Illicit Collaboration

Models of collaboration in which the operating agreement provides the structure and mechanisms that enable morally objectionable procedures to take place at the non-Catholic facility implicate the Catholic institution in implicit formal cooperation. There are different ways in which this can occur. This can happen if the management of the morally objectionable procedures is linked to the executives of the joint entity, for example, if the CEO of the joint entity appoints the CEO of the non-Catholic partner who has management responsibility over the morally objectionable procedures. On the financial side, if an accounting mechanism is agreed to whereby the revenues from morally objectionable procedures are accounted for together with all other revenues from joint operations and then are separated out, the Catholic institution would still be illicitly cooperating in the collection of revenue from the procedures.

Implicit formal cooperation is also possible if the agreement establishes morally objectionable procedures at a former non-Catholic facility now owned and operated by a Catholic institution. Some of the ways in which this can occur is for the Catholic institution to: lease space, utilities, ancillary services, and personnel for the purpose of providing morally objectionable procedures; lease or sell equipment and supplies for the same purpose; ensure that all policies, protocols, procedures, and standards associated with the morally objectionable procedures are consistent with those of the Catholic institution; or assist with the temporary transfer of patients for the purpose of receiving morally objectionable procedures. These same illicit arrangements can also occur with an independent non-Catholic partner.

The National Catholic Bioethics Center recognizes the critical importance of collaborative arrangements between Catholic and non-Catholic health care institutions for the continuation of the Catholic health care ministry. What this and the preceding chapter have shown is that the Catholic moral tradition can be faithfully brought to bear upon the question to produce concrete models of morally acceptable collaboration.

Peter J. Cataldo, Ph.D.
Director of Research
The National Catholic Bioethics Center
Boston, Massachusetts

The Philadelphia Protocol for Collaborative Relationships

Due to the complex nature of health care, some Catholic health care providers have determined that in order to preserve their ministry, there is a pressing need for joint ventures, partnerships, or other types of collaborative relationships relevant to the joint financing and the joint delivery of health care [hereinafter referred to as *Collaborative Relationships*]. It is understood that in such Collaborative Relationships Catholic health care providers operating in the Archdiocese of Philadelphia will give priority to entering into relationships with other Catholic health care institutions and agencies in order that the Catholic presence in the provision of health care might remain strong and influential, witnessing collectively to their shared ministry.

If it is determined that no exclusively Catholic relationship is possible, and a Collaborative Relationship with a non-Catholic provider is proposed, the Catholic health care provider must evaluate the proposed Collaborative Relationship in light of each of the following:

1. The necessity of strengthening the Catholic health care apostolate within the Archdiocese.
2. The future viability of the particular Catholic health care provider as well as the future possible harm to the particular Catholic health care provider if it did not enter into the Collaborative Relationship.
3. The need for pro active advocacy on behalf of Catholic ethical and moral principles.
4. The necessity of avoiding formal cooperation in evil.
5. The necessity to avoid public scandal; and
6. The necessity to educate the community regarding the Collaborative Relationship.

Catholic health care providers shall not enter into any major alliance or affiliation agreement with non-Catholic health care providers without the *nihil obstat* of the Archbishop of Philadelphia. For subsequent "collaborative relationships" flowing from the major alliance or affiliation agreement, a petition for a *nihil obstat* needs to be made only when the Secretary for Catholic Human Services is reasonably concerned that the Collaborative Relationship might negatively affect the mission or religious or ethical identity of such Catholic health care providers.

The Archbishop will specify a process for the review of such ventures in consultation with all relevant parties. Because of the necessity for the Archdiocese to be apprised at the onset, such Collaborative Relationships are to be presented in writing to the Archdiocese of Philadelphia before any substantial negotiations are undertaken with the prospective partners. The Collaborative Relationship will be evaluated in light of church teaching and canonical legislation, the proper law of the sponsors, the necessity of the relationship, and the likely effect that the activity will have on other apostolates within the Archdiocese.

The Archbishop or his delegate will use the following criteria, among others, in evaluating these relationships.

1. Collaborative Relationships shall enhance the local Catholic health care apostolate by:
   a) Helping to implement the church's moral and social teaching.
   b) Furthering the health care ministry to the community.
   c) Witnessing to a responsible stewardship of limited health care resources.
   d) Providing poor and vulnerable persons with a more equitable access to basic health care.
2. All activities arising from the Collaborative Relationship will conform to the *Ethical and Religious Directives for Catholic Health Care Services.*
3. Catholic providers will only enter into Collaborative Relationships that do not violate the principles of cooperation with evil regarding procedures judged to be immoral by the Catholic Church, for example as stated in the *Ethical and Religious Directives for Catholic Health Care Services* as they currently exist or are amended in the future.
4. A Catholic provider cannot own or manage an institution that by policy or practice engages in intrinsically immoral activities.
5. A *nihil obstat* will not be granted to Collaborative Relationships in which the result will be that the Catholic health care provider becomes a publicly traded, investor-owned, for-profit entity so as to lose its not-for-profit status.

The Procedure

Purpose

1. To preserve the Catholic identity and ensure the continuation of the mission of health care apostolates operating within the Archdiocese of Philadelphia.
2. To promote cooperation of all parties involved in the Catholic health care apostolate in the Archdiocese of Philadelphia; and
3. To further the healing ministry that embodies the Gospel message of Jesus Christ as reflected in the values and teachings of the Catholic Church and in the *Ethical and Religious Directives for Catholic Health Care Services*.

Scope

In compliance with particular law of the Archdiocese of Philadelphia, promulgated February 25, 1999, and effective as of March 25, 1999, all Catholic health care providers operating in the Archdiocese are obligated to follow these procedures.

Policy

1. The Archbishop of Philadelphia shall establish the Catholic Health Care Review Committee ("*Committee*").
2. This Committee will review all proposed Collaborative Relationships with non-Catholic providers which would result in a major alliance or affiliation and thereby require the *nihil obstat* of the Archbishop of Philadelphia. For subsequent Collaborative Relationships flowing from the major alliance or affiliation agreement, or other Collaborative Relationships of a less substantive nature, review by the Committee will only occur upon recommendation from the Secretary for Catholic Human Services.
3. The Committee will provide a recommendation to the Archbishop of Philadelphia regarding the appropriateness of such Collaborative Relationships based on the criteria defined in the relevant particular law.
4. The Committee will consist of the Secretary for Catholic Human Services of the Archdiocese of Philadelphia (who will serve as chair), no more than three priests, one member of a religious congregation, and one Catholic layperson, all of whom will have some expertise in Catholic health care issues.
5. The members of the Committee shall be appointed to serve for a term of three years, which may be renewed once.
6. The Archbishop shall appoint all the members of the Committee.
7. The Committee will have the opportunity for consultation with indi-

viduals or appropriate recognized groups with the requisite expertise in civil law, canon law, moral theology, and health care.

Procedure

The procedure for the evaluation of Collaborative Relationships which affect the mission or religious and ethical identity of Catholic health care providers is as follows:

1. Because of the necessity for the Archdiocese to be apprised at the onset, the health care provider will notify in writing the Secretary for Catholic Human Services of the potential for such a Collaborative Relationship before any substantial negotiations are undertaken with the prospective partner. In consultation with the Catholic health care provider, the Secretary will either monitor the proposal, ask for additional information , or refer the proposal to the Committee. Prior to the submission of any proposal to the Committee, the Secretary will work with the Catholic health care provider to assure that the draft which is to be reviewed reflects all changes which have been recommended by the appropriate consultants.
2. In collaboration with the Catholic health care provider proposing the Collaborative Relationship, the Committee will determine the time line necessary for submission to the Archbishop for his consideration. While it is understood that the Committee will always be sensitive to the time constraints of the Catholic health care provider, it is likewise noted that the Committee itself will require adequate time to read and evaluate the documents submitted to it.
3. The Committee will determine the extent of the review based on the significance and nature of the matter.
4. Upon completion of its review, the Committee will submit its report and a recommendation to the Archbishop for his consideration.
5. All Committee discussions, meetings, correspondence, and recommendations to the Archbishop are to be maintained in the strictest confidence.
6. The procedure will be reviewed after three years. The Secretary for Catholic Human Services will initiate this review.

The Archdiocese of Philadelphia
Philadelphia, Pennsylvania

Five Principles for Collaborative Arrangements

The following are the five principles (sometimes called the "Smith" principles, in honor of the Rev. Russell Smith) are used at The National Catholic Bioethics Center for evaluating the collaborative arrangements of Catholic health care facilities with non-Catholic partners. The Center has analyzed a great number of these contractual arrangements over its twenty-five year history. The principles summarize that experience and provide what we believe to be the most effective means of preserving the identity of Catholic health care.

1. *We can only do together what all partners agree to be appropriate. The collaborative venture need not be Catholic, but it must observe the* Ethical and Religious Directives (*or some secular version thereof*) *out of respect for the corporate conscience of the Catholic partner.*
2. *Cooperation must be mediate material, never formal or immediate material.*
3. *Morally illicit procedures cannot be provided on the Catholic campus.*
4. *Any morally illicit procedures on the campuses of non-Catholic partners must be excluded from the new alliance by separate incorporation and separate billing mechanisms.*
5. *Publicity concerning the collaborative venture should explain the necessity of the alliance for the sake of the Catholic health care apostolate; describe the financial and other goods achieved through the alliance; and note the exclusion of immoral procedures from the partnership (though they remain available through the partner operating under its own auspices)* .

The Ethicists
The National Catholic Bioethics Center
Boston, Massachusetts

Index

A

abortion 12, 83, 134, 140, 141, 145, 148; hiring providers 130–132; as intrinsic evil 77; and public life 27–30, 127.
absolutes, moral 6, 21–22
amputation 89
anger 57
anthropology, Christian 49–52, 63–65
Aquinas, St. Thomas 7, 25, 37–39, 51, 57, 73, 115–117; on human acts 34, 82, 143; on mutilation 85, 89; on natural law 41–43, 128
Aristotle 24, 53, 128; on teleology 49–51, 81–82; on virtue; 15, 39, 115–117
Ashley, Benedict 65, 86
Augustine, St. Aurelius 34, 51, 56, 116
authority 35
autonomy 8, 42, 63–66; false 26, 51, 64

B

Bañez, Domingo 89
baptism 84
Beatitudes 35
beauty 42, 55
Bernardin, Joseph 100
bioethics 37–40
bishop, role of 105, 151–154
Browne, Sir Thomas 59
Buddha 54

C

capital 98, 149
Catechism of the Catholic Church 7, 15, 19, 88, 115; on moral acts 73–77, 81
charity 9, 15, 19, 75, 111
charity care 98–99
Chesterton, G.K. 54
choice 74
chorioamnionitis 83
Christ [see Jesus Christ]
Cicero 41, 127
circumstances 67, 69, 73, 77, 90, and cooperation 140–141, 143; and double effect 81–83
code, medical 11; Nuremburg 120–121
collaborative ventures, corporate 135, 139–146, 147–150, 151–154
Commandments, Ten [Decalogue] 7, 21, 35, 37–38, 41, 50
committee, ethics [see ethics committee]
commutative justice 117
compassion 13–16, 60; virtue of 15
condoms 12
confidentiality 111–114
conscience 23–26, 38, 43, 103, 106; and Church teaching 20, 41, 77, 155
consent, informed 88, 103, 120–122
consent and morality 127
consequences 67, 71
consequentialism 67
contemplation 50
contraception 68–71, 140
cooperation 8, 130–132, 133–136, 139–146, 147–150, 152; continuous 145; formal 134, 140–141, 145–150, 151, 155, material 134, 141, 143, 145, 148, 155
Corwin, Edward 128
counsel [taking advice] 25
creation 116–117

D

Dark Night of the Soul [St. John of the Cross] 58
Darwin, Charles 116

death, culture of 13, 15
death with dignity 5
Decalogue [see Commandments, Ten]
Declaration on Euthanasia 91
Dei Filius 21
Dei Verbum 19
Dignitatis humanae 20
dignity, human 13, 97, 105–108, 114, 139, 146; as Catholic principle 5–8, 85, 121–122, 129
dignity, loss of 16
disorder, intrinsic 6
dissent 22, 36, 70–71
distributive justice 117
divorce 33
dominion 63–66
Donne, John 25
Donum vitae 76
double effect, principle of 8, 69, 81–84, 87, 90
doubt, Cartesian 24
duress 142–145
duty, ethics of 37–40

E

education 39, 54, 105–106
embryo, frozen 145–146
end, intended 73–77
end, of medicine 101–102, 104
Enlightenment 37, 127
Ethical and Religious Directives for Catholic Health Care Services, on cooperation 134, 139, 142, 147–149, 152–153; on ethics committees 105–108; on human dignity 5–8; on human experimentation 122; on human suffering 59; as moral norm for Catholic health care 10, 136, 146; on pregnancy 84; on principle of integrity 86–88; on service to others 97; on stewardship 65
ethics committee 105–108
ethics, situation 71
euthanasia 5, 76–77, 91–92, 140, 145
Evangelium vitae 13, 64
evil, intrinsic 21–22, 67–71, 74, 77, 133–135, 143, 145, 152; "lesser" 133; premoral 43, 67–71
ex cathedra 21
excellence, human 5, 6
ex integra causa 75
experimentation, human 119–122
extraordinary means [see means, ordinary vs. extraordinary]

F

faith and morals 19–21
faith and reason 51, 108
Fall, the 52
flourishing, human 23
formal cooperation (see cooperation, formal)
freedom and truth 24
freedom, human 27, 35, 41–43, 133
freedom, moral 38, 65

G

Gaudium et spes 20, 63–65, 85–86
Genesis 64
God 6; as Creator 49, 64, 103, 108; design of 65; as end 38; *Logos,* 56; person as image of 6, 8, 12; sovereignty of 15
good, common 99, 106, 108, 111, 112, 117; health as 102; hierarchy of 7; human 74–76, 81; intrinsic 74; knowledge of 10–11; social 97
government, democracy 23; divine 42–43
grace 50–51
Griese, Orville 112
Grisez, Germain 21

H

Hamlet 24
happiness, pursuit of 49–52
health care, non-profit 97–100
health, end of medicine 102
Helsinki Declaration 120
Hobbes, Thomas 53, 116
Holmes, Oliver Wendell 126
hope 58, 60
horror, psychological 89–90
human acts, principles of 34
human subjects, research on 119–122
Humanae vitae 70
Hume, David 14

I

identity, Catholic 9–12, 153, 155
illusion 57–58
Incarnation 55–56
inclinations, natural 38–39, 42, 82, 116
infallibility 19–21
insemination, artificial 145
integrity of the body 85–88, 89
intention, 73–77,140, 145; and double effect 81–84,
investor-owned health care 97–100
in vitro fertilization 7, 76–77, 145–146
informed consent 8
intrinsic evil (see evil, intrinsic)

J

Jesus Christ, imitation of 19, 35, 43, 114, 146; suffering of 58–59; teachings of 41, 50, 53–56, 144, 153
Job 57–58, 64
John of the Cross, St. 58
John Paul II, Pope, on the good of human life 13, 16; on human dignity 85, 114; on human suffering and compassion 59; moral teaching of 19–20, 34-35, 50, 71; on the natural law 34, 41-43; on reevangelizing the world 144;
joint ventures [see collaborative ventures]
judgment, moral 20, 25
jurisprudence, sociological 125–126
justice 27–28, 111, 128, 144; social virtue of 115–118

K

Kant, Immanuel 39, 50, 54–55, 63, 127
Keenan, James 81
Kevorkian, Jack 12
killing (human beings) 27–30

L

labor, early induction 83–84
law, and authority 33; civil 41; eternal 20, 41–42; and grace 34; and morality 28, 38–39, 41–43, 75, 77, 125–128; natural 33–36, 39, 41–43, 75, 103, 115, 117, 125–128; New 41, 43, 55–56; positive 33–34, 125, 127–128; and virtue 36
Lear, King 57, 60
legalism, moral 7, 54
Lehmkuhl, Augustinus 89
Leo XIII, Pope 41
liberty [see freedom]
life, purpose of 10, 49; quality of 14–15; sanctity of 15
life support, removal of 91
ligations, tubal 7, 12, 86, 134 (see also sterilization)
Ligouri, Alphonsus 133
Lind, James 119
luck 51
Lumen Gentium 21, 66

M

MacIntyre, Alasdair, 37
malpractice 112
manuals [see tradition, manualist]
Magisterium 19–22, 36, 67–70, 91, 146
Marxism 116
masturbation 68–70
material cooperation (see cooperation, material)
McCormick, Richard 67–71
means, ordinary vs. extraordinary 8, 89–92
medical care, free 9
medical records 114
medicine, goal of 11–12; as cognitive art 102; computerized 112; as knowledge 102
"medspeak" 114
memories, repressed 113
Meno [Plato] 53
moral object (see object, moral)
moral presuppositions 11
moral quality 73
morality, imposing on others 27–30
mutilation 85–86, 89, 121

N

nature, human 74, 82, 84
Nicomachean Ethics 81
Nietzsche, Friedrich 37
nihil obstat 151–153
nominalism 127
non-profit health care 97–100, 152

O

Oath, Hippocratic 11, 111
object, moral 67–69, 71, 73–77, 81–83, 133, 140–142
organ donation 87–88
orientation, sexual 113
O'Rourke, Kevin 65, 86

P

pain 89–90
Paul, St. 53, 58
Pellegrino, Edmund 63, 102
perfection, Christian 50, 58
person, human 29, 43, 103–104
philosophers, pre-Christian 115
philosophy, modern 127; moral 34, 36
physician-assisted suicide 5, 140, 145–146
physican-patient relationship 106, 108, 114
Pinckaers, Servais 37–39, 82
Pius XII, Pope 86, 90, 121
Planned Parenthood v. *Casey* 33
Plato 49, 53, 115–116
pluralism 27
principles 55–56; *a priori* 54–55; cooperation 133–136, 139–146, 152; first 25
probabilism 38
pro-life 27–30
proportionalism 67–71, 91
protocol, collaborative 151–154
prudence 25, 77, 82–84, 118; improper 34, 36

Q

Quinlan, Karen 107

R

Rahner, Karl 21
Ratzinger, Joseph Cardinal 23–24
realism, legal 125–126
reason, human 41–43, 127–128; practical 82; right 70, 89; sufficient 134–135; "why" 74, 82
records, medical 114
redemption 6, 59
Reformation 37
relationships, collaborative (see collaborative ventures)

relativism 54, 128–129
Renaissance 89, 127
Republic, of Cicero 41; of Plato 115
resuscitation 91
revelation, divine 43, 50, 115
right, human 49, 117–118, 120–121; as confidentiality 111; and natural law 41–42
Roe v. *Wade* 126
Rousseau, Jean-Jacques 14, 53, 116

S

saints, the 55
salvation 50–51, 58
Salvifici doloris 59
scandal 133–135, 147–148, 151
science 66; authority of 10, 108; and research 119–122; social 126; and technology 101–103
scientism 101
"selective reduction" 11
self-knowledge 57; self-love 75; self-preservation 42
sentiment, as basis of morality 13, 15, 55–56, 117
Sermon on the Mount 41
Shakespeare 24, 57, 60
Shannon, Thomas 63
Simon, Yves 35–36
sin 7, 144; punishment for 57
Sinai, Mount 43, 50
Spirit, Holy 43
sterilization 68–70, 77, 87, 145
stewardship 63–66, 152
Stoicism 50, 57, 128
subjectivity, relativistic 23
suffering 5, 13–16; and conversion 58; mystery of 57–60
Summa contra Gentiles 115
Summa Theologiae 25, 37–39, 57, 82, 85, 89, 115–117, 143
Supreme Court, U.S. 125
surrogacy 11
synderesis 25

T

technology 66; limits of 59; medical 101–104
teleology 49–51, 65, 103–104
theology, moral 37–38, 89, 133; and authority 33, contemporary 36, 64; and proportionalism 67–71
theology, speculative 39
Tocqueville, Alexis de 127
tradition, Aristotelian-Thomistic 37; Cartesian 43; Catholic 19, 21, 71, 75; classical 25; manualist 37–40, 41; rationalistic 37
Trent, Council of 37
truth 23–24; telling the 111–114
tubal ligations (see ligations, tubal)

U

unborn, the 27–30, 125
uninsured patients 99–100
utilitarianism 28

V

Values Statement, Common 147–149
vasectomies 7
Vatican Council, Second 19–21, 64, 66
Veritatis splendor 19–21, 23, 24, 34, 41, 43, 50, 65, 67, 73, 77, 81, 85, 133
virtue, 50–51, 53, 115–118; ethics 33–36, 37, habits of 38, 116

W

Weber, Max 126
William of Occam 37, 127
willing 74–76